Environment, Health and Sustainable Development

Understanding Public Health Series

Series editors: Nicki Thorogood and Rosalind Plowman, London School of Hygiene & Tropical Medicine (previous edition edited by Nick Black and Rosalind Raine)

Throughout the world, recognition of the importance of public health to sustainable, safe and healthy societies is growing. The achievements of public health in nineteenth-century Europe were for much of the twentieth century overshadowed by advances in personal care, in particular in hospital care. Now, with the dawning of a new century, there is increasing understanding of the inevitable limits of individual health care and of the need to complement such services with effective public health strategies. Major improvements in people's health will come from controlling communicable diseases, eradicating environmental hazards, improving people's diets, and enhancing the availability and quality of effective health care. To achieve this, every country needs a cadre of knowledgeable public health practitioners with social, political and organizational skills to lead and bring about changes at international, national and local levels. This is one of a series of books that provides a foundation for those wishing to join in and contribute to the twenty-first-century regeneration of public health, helping to put the concerns and perspectives of public health at the heart of policy-making and service provision. While each book stands alone, together they provide a comprehensive account of the three main aims of public health: protecting the public from environmental hazards, improving the health of the public and ensuring high-quality health services are available to all. Some of the books focus on methods, others on key topics. They have been written by staff at the London School of Hygiene & Tropical Medicine with considerable experience of teaching public health to students from low-, middle- and high-income countries. Much of the material has been developed and tested with postgraduate students both in face-to-face teaching and through distance learning.

The books are designed for self-directed learning. Each chapter has explicit learning objectives, key terms are highlighted and the text contains many activities to enable the reader to test their own understanding of the ideas and material covered. Written in a clear and accessible style, the series will be essential reading for students taking postgraduate courses in public health and will also be of interest to public health practitioners and policy-makers.

Titles in the series

Analytical models for decision making: Colin Sanderson and Reinhold Gruen
Conflict and health: Natasha Howard, Egbert Sondorp and Annemarie Ter Veen (eds)
Controlling communicable disease: Norman Noah
Economic analysis for management and policy: Stephen Jan, Lilani Kumaranayake, Jenny Roberts, Kara Hanson and Kate Archibald
Economic evaluation: Julia Fox-Rushby and John Cairns (eds)
Environmental epidemiology: Paul Wilkinson (ed.)
Environmental health policy: Megan Landon and Tony Fletcher
Financial management in health services: Reinhold Gruen and Anne Howarth
Globalization and health, second edition: Johanna Hanefeld (ed.)
Health care evaluation: Sarah Smith, Don Sinclair, Rosalind Raine and Barnaby Reeves
Health promotion theory, second edition: Liza Cragg, Maggie Davies and Wendy MacDowall (eds)
Health promotion practice, second edition: Will Nutland and Liza Cragg (eds)
Introduction to epidemiology, second edition: Ilona Carneiro and Natasha Howard
Introduction to health economics, second edition: Lorna Guinness and Virginia Wiseman (eds)
Issues in public health, second edition: Fiona Sim and Martin McKee (eds)
Making health policy, second edition: Kent Buse, Nicholas Mays and Gill Walt
Managing health services: Nick Goodwin, Reinhold Gruen and Valerie Iles
Medical anthropology: Robert Pool and Wenzel Geissler
Principles of social research, second edition: Mary Alison Durand and Tracey Chantler (eds)
Public health in history: Virginia Berridge, Martin Gorsky and Alex Mold
Sexual health: A public health perspective: Kay Wellings, Kirstin Mitchell and Martine Collumbien (eds)
Understanding health services: Nick Black and Reinhold Gruen

Forthcoming titles

Applied communicable disease control, Gregory Thomas-Reilly, Liza Cragg and Will Nutland
Health care evaluation, second edition, Carmen Tsang and David Cromwell (eds)
Understanding health services, second edition, İpek Gürol-Urgancı, Fiona Campbell and Nick Black

Environment, Health and Sustainable Development

Second edition

Edited by Emma Hutchinson and
Sari Kovats

 Open University Press

Open University Press
McGraw-Hill Education
8th Floor
338 Euston Road
London
NW1 3BH

email: enquiries@openup.co.uk
world wide web: www.mheducation.co.uk

and Two Penn Plaza, New York, NY 10121-2289, USA

First published 2006
First published in this second edition 2016

A catalogue record of this book is available from the British Library

ISBN-13: 978-0-33-524537-6
ISBN-10: 0-33-524537-4
eISBN: 978-0-33-524538-3

Library of Congress Cataloging-in-Publication Data
CIP data applied for

Typeset by Transforma Pvt. Ltd., Chennai, India
Printed and bound by CPI Group (UK) Ltd, Croydon, CRO 4YY

Praise for this book

"The fully revised second edition presents the wide range of environmental issues that are relevant to public health with academic rigour, but loses none of the ease of use for self-directed study of the first edition, with several new activities and feedback within each chapter."

Dr Sotiris Vardoulakis, Head of Environmental
Change Department, Public Health England, UK

"The broadening of the traditional scope of environmental health is clearly presented in this book. The 19th century view of this branch of public health still prevalent among public health practitioners has finally been updated, with a change to a global perspective. Energy choices, climate change, ecosystem services, waste are now appropriately included as environmental factors affecting health, and through this lens traditional topics of air, water and soil can be re-interpreted. This overview provides a solid foundation for all public health practitioners intending to include environmental health as part of a renewed mainstream public health capable of engaging with the full range of environmental challenges to sustainable health and wellbeing in contemporary societies."

Giovanni Leonardi, Head of the Environmental
Epidemiology Group, Public Health England, UK

Contents

List of figures, tables and boxes

Figures

Tables

Boxes

List of authors

ARACELI BUSBY is a consultant in health protection for Public Health England, UK.

EMMA HUTCHINSON is a lecturer at the London School of Hygiene & Tropical Medicine, UK, and module organizer of environment, health and sustainable development on the distance learning MSc programme in public health.

MARIA-JOSE LOPEZ-ESPINOSA is at the Foundation for the Promotion of Health and Biomedical Research in the Valencian Region, FISABIO-Public Health, Valencia, Spain.

SARI KOVATS is a senior lecturer at the London School of Hygiene & Tropical Medicine, UK, and director of the NIHR Health Protection Research Unit in Environmental Change and Health.

JAMES MILNER is a lecturer at the London School of Hygiene & Tropical Medicine, UK, and module organizer of environmental health policy on the distance learning MSc programme in public health.

DEBAPRIYA MONDAL is an environmental toxicologist at the School of Environmental and Life Sciences, University of Salford, UK.

VIRGINIA MURRAY is a consultant in global disaster risk reduction at Public Health England, and vice-chair of the Science and Technical Advisory Group of UNISDR (United Nations Office for Disaster Risk Reduction).

RACHEL PELETZ is director of programmes at the Aquaya Institute, Kenya.

NOAH SCOVRONICK is a postdoctoral research associate at Princeton University, USA, where he is affiliated with the Climate Futures Initiative and the Woodrow Wilson School.

CATHRYN TONNE is an environmental epidemiologist at CREAL (Centre for Research in Environmental Epidemiology) in Barcelona, Spain.

CAROLYN STEPHENS is visiting full professor of ecology and global health at the Faculty of Medicine of the National University of Tucumán (UNT), Argentina, and honorary full professor at the UCL Institute of Health Equity, UK.

Acknowledgements

The editors would like to thank the contributors past and present, involved in the course taught at LSHTM, for providing lecture notes and references as a basis for the book, specifically, Tony Fletcher, Joeren Ensink, Paul Wilkinson, David Satterthwaite, Kristie Ebi, Peter Baxter, Mike Joffe, Ben Armstrong, Sandy Cairncross, Virginia Berridge, Alex Mold, Shakoor Hajat, Angela Mawle, and David Pencheon, and chapter authors Maria-Jose Lopez-Espinosa, Debapriya Mondal, Rachel Peletz, James Milner, Cathryn Tonne, Noah Scovronick, Araceli Busby, Virginia Murray and Carolyn Stephens.

Helpful editorial comments on chapters were provided by Ben Armstrong, Paul Wilkinson, Sandy Cairncross, Costas Velis, Steven Cummins, Jason Vargo, Simon Lloyd, Susannah Mayhew and Ruth Willis, and the series editors Rosalind Plowman and Nicki Thorogood. We also thank Megan Landon who wrote the first edition of this book.

Emma Hutchinson would also like to thank her children, Calum, Bethan, Rafi and Cai, and her partner, Paul for their continued support while editing and contributing to writing this book.

Sari Kovats would like to thank Willow, Joseph, and Graham for their support and patience.

Overview of the book

Introduction

Environmental health is the branch of public health concerned with assessing and understanding the impact of the environment on people. This book has three sections – the first is an introduction to the concepts of environment, health and sustainable development, and the frameworks used to assess how these relate to each other. The second section explores in more detail the environmental hazards that affect health (chemicals, water and sanitation, air pollution, transport, waste, the built environment, disasters, climate change and the natural environment). The third section looks at actions to address these environmental hazards. Each chapter uses examples from low-, middle- and high-income countries. We do not attempt to cover the effects of environment on agriculture or nutrition in this book.

Why study environmental health and sustainable development?

The overall aim of this book is to show how health is related to the environment, and further to improve understanding of environmental issues in public health policy and practice. Its objectives are:

1 To demonstrate the links between health, environment and sustainable development.
2 To explain equity and sustainability as central principles in public health.
3 To describe the health effects of key environmental hazards.
4 To assess the health implications of global environmental change, including the urban transition, climate change and loss of ecosystem services.
5 To evaluate how environmental issues are addressed in current public health practice, and to understand mechanisms for policy action.

Structure of the book

This book follows the conceptual outline of the 'Environment, health and sustainable development' module taught at the London School of Hygiene & Tropical Medicine. It is based on the materials presented in the lectures and seminars of the taught course, which have been adapted for distance learning. Each chapter includes:

- an overview;
- a list of learning objectives;
- a list of key terms;
- a range of activities;
- feedback on the activities;
- a summary.

The following description of the book sections will give an idea of what is covered in each section. There is also a glossary at the end of the book to help with unfamiliar terms.

Section 1: Introduction and concepts

Chapter 1 introduces the concepts underlying the book – health, environment and sustainable development – and how these relate to environmental justice and health inequalities. Humans experience a wide range of social and environmental determinants that affect health. Frameworks for linking environment with human health are discussed in Chapter 2. Mechanisms for exposure to hazards are described and an introduction to risk assessment – used to estimate the effect of environmental factors on health – is presented. The chapter concludes with a consideration of what constitutes a healthy environment. Chapter 3 focuses on environmental change – how human activities cause environmental problems through emissions of pollutants, resource depletion and environmental degradation. This chapter discusses the transitions that are important for public health (demographic, epidemiological, urban, technological, energy). The chapter briefly discusses some policy objectives to reduce the impacts of humans on the environment, such as the Sustainable Development Goals (SDGs).

Section 2: Environmental hazards

Environmental hazards are explored using examples from populations in high-, middle- and low-income countries. The hazards include chemicals, biological contamination (relating to water and sanitation), the indoor environment, housing, outdoor air pollution, transport and waste.

Chapter 4 explores the impact on health of chemicals in the environment (in air, water and soil). Chapter 5 explores the relationship of water and sanitation to health. Many of us spend most of our time indoors. Chapter 6 introduces the hazards of the indoor environment: the effect of cold homes and the burden of indoor air pollution from biomass fuels. Outdoor air pollution is a significant environmental health problem in nearly all countries and is discussed in Chapter 7. Road transport is a major contributor to urban outdoor air pollution and also affects health through traffic accidents. Chapter 8 considers the health implications of different methods of solid waste disposal, particularly landfill and incineration.

In Chapter 9, we address the environmental health issues associated with the urban environment, and how cities can be designed to improve the health of their inhabitants. Chapter 10 discusses the health consequences of natural and technological disasters. We also consider the role of public health in disaster prevention, preparedness and response. In Chapter 11, health effects of the different methods of energy generation are described, including biomass and fossil fuel combustion, and nuclear power and hydro-electric power. Chapter 12 covers the impact on health of climate variability and the difficulties in assessing the future health consequences of global climate change. The effects on health from stratospheric ozone depletion are also discussed. Chapter 13 considers the concept of ecosystem services and how the natural environment provides benefits for human health.

Section 3: Policy

The final chapter focuses on environment and health policy at local, national and international levels. Chapter 14 provides a brief overview of local, national and international environmental policy-making, how this can benefit public health and the role that public health can play in policy-making. The chapter explores the importance of local plans for sustainable development, as well as international environmental agreements. It also discusses how policies can be developed to address both health and environmental objectives.

SECTION 1

Introduction and concepts

Introduction

Emma Hutchinson

Overview

Where people live and work is their environment. It encompasses their surroundings and includes physical, biological, social, cultural and economic factors. People constantly interact with their environment: it helps shape their lives and it affects their health. A poor quality environment is responsible for a significant proportion of the global burden of disease. The aim of this chapter is to encourage thinking about how environment and health are related, and how these relate to your own experiences and circumstances. Sustainable development will be introduced as a concept and we will explore how this is related to health, and how healthy communities can be achieved by adhering to the underlying principles of sustainable development.

Learning objectives

By the end of this chapter you will be able to:

- understand the relationships between human activities, human health and the environment
- understand the concepts of environmental health inequalities and inequity
- appraise the concept of sustainable development

Key terms

Environment: Physical, biological and social conditions affecting people's lives.

Environmental health: Those aspects of human health, including quality of life, that are determined by physical, biological, economic and cultural factors in the environment. It also refers to the theory and practice of assessing, correcting, controlling and preventing these factors in the environment that potentially can adversely affect the health of present and future generations.

Health inequalities: Differences in health experience and health status between countries, regions and socioeconomic or social groups.

Health inequities: *Avoidable* inequalities in health between groups of people within countries and between countries.

Sustainable development: Development that meets the needs of the present, without compromising the ability of future generations to meet their own needs.

Environment, health, and sustainable development

The quality of the environment is an important determinant of health. Biological agents in the environment such as parasites and pathogens are a cause of illness and premature death for millions of people in the developing world. Outdoor and household air pollution also affect the health of millions.

Historically, economic development has often been accompanied by environmental degradation and resource depletion (WHO 2006). In order to achieve a balance between improving human health and wellbeing and protecting the environment, it is desirable for development to be made sustainable by achieving *both* the following objectives:

- economic development to meet people's needs (food, shelter, water, security, access to health care, education, employment, etc.);
- ecological sustainability to ensure that natural resources can be sustained for present and future use without being irreparably damaged or destroyed.

Sustainable development is therefore about more than just the environment, it is also about ensuring a strong, healthy and just society.

What is health?

The World Health Organization (WHO) defines health as the state of complete physical, mental and social wellbeing and not merely the absence of disease or infirmity (WHO 1948). The conditions required for good health include sufficient resources to meet basic human needs (such as food and water), and protection from environmental hazards.

The WHO was instrumental in producing and promoting a charter for health promotion (the Ottawa Charter for Health Promotion) that encompasses the component parts of health and recommended action designed to achieve 'Health for All' (WHO 1986). The Charter states that in order to achieve a state of complete physical, mental and social wellbeing, individuals or groups must be able to identify and to realize aspirations, to satisfy needs, and to change or cope with the environment. The fundamental conditions and resources for health are: peace; shelter; education; food; income; a stable ecosystem; sustainable resources; social justice; and equity (WHO 1986).

What is the environment?

The environment can be considered to be everything around us, or more specifically, all external (i.e. non-genetic) factors: physical, biological, social, economic and cultural (Frumkin 2010). The impact of the environment is more than just that of individual hazards affecting health (such as air pollutants), but also the effect of less easily measurable conditions such as the quality of our neighbourhood. See Chapter 2 for more discussion of environment and how we measure its impact.

Environmental effects range from the local (air pollution, water pollution, waste) to the regional (forest fires, transboundary air pollution), to those on a global scale (climate change). These topics are covered in depth in Chapters 4–8 (chemicals, water, indoor and outdoor air quality and waste) and Chapters 12 and 13 (global climate systems and ecosystem services).

Environmental health

The WHO defines environmental health as those aspects of human health, including quality of life, that are determined by physical, biological, social also cultural and economic factors in the environment. These relationships and their interactions are illustrated in Figure 1.1. Environmental health also refers to the theory and practice of assessing, correcting, controlling and preventing those factors in the environment that potentially can adversely affect the health of present and future generations (WHO 1993).

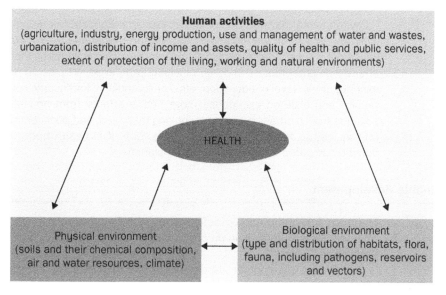

Figure 1.1 Interaction between human activities and the physical and biological environment.
Source: Adapted from WHO (1992).

The links between humans and their environment suggest that an inter-sectoral approach to health is advisable in order to maintain good health. Health is not only the responsibility of doctors, nurses and other medical personnel, but should also be considered the responsibility of non-health agencies who have the knowledge and power to change the environment, and therefore affect the health of the population at large.

The WHO states that 'the overall guiding principle for the world, nations, regions and communities alike, is the need to encourage reciprocal maintenance – to take care of each other, our communities and our natural environment' (WHO 2010). Therefore, the conservation of natural resources throughout the world can be seen as a global responsibility. Not all subscribe to this view, however, and this is explored further in Chapter 14, Activity 14.3.

Inequalities and inequity in health

It is important to distinguish between inequality in health and inequity. Health inequalities can be defined as differences in health status or in the distribution of health determinants between different population groups (WHO 2016). Some health inequalities are attributable to biological variations or free choice and others are attributable to the external environment outside the control of the individuals concerned. In the first case, it may be impossible or ethically or ideologically unacceptable to change the health determinants and so the health inequalities are unavoidable. In the second, the uneven distribution may be unnecessary and avoidable as well as unjust and unfair, so that the resulting health inequalities also lead to inequity in health (WHO 2016).

Environmental hazards do not affect everyone equally. Some individuals (children, people on low incomes) may be more vulnerable to environmental causes of disease than others. Social factors which can increase the impact of environmental factors on health include living in poverty, being part of a minority group, level of education, etc. For example, in low-income countries, women and children experience more health effects from household air pollution from biomass burning for cooking than men, and poor communities with access to few resources bear the burden of ill health from biomass burning compared to higher income populations.

Sustainable development

The most frequently quoted definition of sustainable development is that from the World Commission on Environment and Development, given in the Brundtland Report:

'sustainable development is development that meets the needs of the present generation without compromising the ability of future generations to meet their own needs' (WHO 1987).

The UK Sustainable Development Commission has provided a useful and succinct explanation:

> *The concept of sustainable development can be interpreted in many different ways, but at its core is an approach to development that looks to balance different, and often competing, needs against an awareness of the environmental, social and economic limitations we face as a society.*
> (SDC 2011)

Throughout our history, humans have interacted with the environment and freely used natural resources. It is only now that we are beginning to understand that there are long-term consequences that can result from the unrestricted use and abuse of the environment. It is this that the principles of sustainable development aim to address. Sustainable development aims to sustain economic development while respecting an environmental and social balance, at all scales, from local to global, and over time.

Environmental justice and sustainable development

Sustainable development is also about addressing inequity within the present generation. It is often the poorest groups in society who are most exposed to environmental hazards, including dangerous working conditions and restricted access to adequate shelter and safe food and water. In addition, these groups are often those with the least access to resources to address this. The importance of addressing this kind of inequity has been enshrined as part of the United Nations Universal Declaration of Human Rights since 1948: 'all people have the right to a standard of living adequate for the health and well-being of themselves and their family, including food, clothing, housing, health care and the necessary social services'.

It is only relatively recently, however, that this declaration has been translated into action that will aim to ensure these rights for present and future generations. Building on the work of the landmark Rio Earth Summit in 1992 (UN Conference on Environment and Development), it is now understood that for development to be sustainable it must not only generate wealth, it must also advance social justice, reduce and eventually eliminate poverty, and remain within the limits imposed by ecosystem and resource resilience (IISD 2012).

A 'common vision' for sustainable development was set out and agreed at the Rio+20 Earth Summit held in Rio de Janeiro, Brazil, from 20–22 June 2012 (UNSDC 2012). This illustrates the various conditions which ideally need to be met to achieve sustainable development, and focused on:

> *... poverty eradication, changing unsustainable and promoting sustainable patterns of consumption and production, and protecting and managing the natural resource base of economic and social development...*

promoting sustained, inclusive and equitable economic growth, creating greater opportunities for all, reducing inequalities, raising basic standards of living; fostering equitable social development and inclusion; and promoting integrated and sustainable management of natural resources and eco-systems that supports inter alia economic, social and human development while facilitating ecosystem conservation, regeneration and restoration and resilience in the face of new and emerging challenges.

While consideration of these broader aspects is useful to help our understanding of the concept of sustainable development, the main aspects focused on in this book are the physical and biological aspects of environment, how these impact on health and how sustainable development relates to these. The concept of environmental justice is discussed further in Chapter 2.

Development of frameworks for sustainable development

Traditionally, sustainable development has been considered to be comprised of 'three pillars': environmental, economic and social objectives (Kemp and Parto 2005). Sometimes culture and politics are also recognized as distinct objectives, with culture increasingly gaining status as the 'fourth pillar' (UCLG 2010). This approach has been useful in highlighting the links between desirable social, economic and environmental qualities and in illustrating that much of our current practice is not sustainable. However, the approach has been subject to criticism as the tendency to consider the 'three pillars' separately has proved hard to overcome and has resulted in continued separation of social, economic and ecological analyses, rather than also addressing areas of overlap and interdependency (Lehtonen 2004; Kemp and Parto 2005). Alternative depictions stressing interconnections and consideration of institutional aspects have been suggested to address these criticisms (Lehtonen 2004; Spangenberg and Giljum 2005).

The relationship between public health and sustainable development is being increasingly recognized. Sustainable development and health are closely interrelated in several ways (UNCED 1992; WHO 1992).

- First, the concept of sustainable development embraces environmental, social and economic dimensions and aspires to health-enhancing communities, societies and environments.
- Second, health is determined by a range of environmental, social and economic influences, and therefore the health of people, places and the planet are interdependent.
- Third, the causes of unsustainable development and poor health are often the same.

A good example of a strategy for how sustainable development can potentially produce healthy societies is available from the UK. The UK adopted a national 'Sustainable Development Strategy' which endorsed the UN

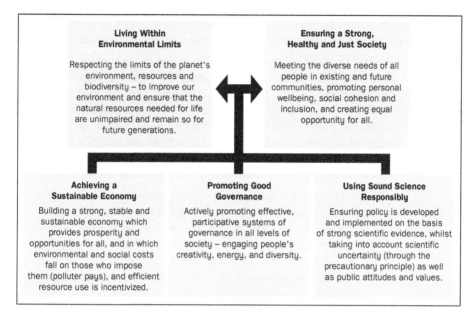

Figure 1.2 UK Sustainable Development Commission: five guiding principles for sustainable development.

definition (see above) and outlined five further guiding principles: living within environmental limits; ensuring a strong, healthy and just society; achieving a sustainable economy; using sound science responsibly; and promoting good governance. These are illustrated in Figure 1.2. Essentially, the framework suggests that by following these principles, we can ensure that resources needed for life will be available now and in future generations (HM Government 2005).

Activity 1.1

You have now been introduced to the definitions of health, the environment and sustainable development, as used in this book. The aim of this activity is for you to use what you have learnt to extend your thinking about how these areas might be integrated.

1 What are the relationships between human activities, human health and sustainable development?
2 Can you outline some of the differences in the patterns of health and disease between low-, middle- and high-income countries? What do you think are the reasons for these differences?
3 Can you think of any differences between men and women in their relationship to the environment?

Feedback

In order to make long-term economic progress and improve health, it is important to consider the environment, health and sustainable development together. For example, it is difficult to make progress on the economic growth of a community if the water supply is inadequate for essential needs. Likewise, economic development and social growth will be impeded if communities are living in informal settlements on the urban fringe, subjected to environmental degradation and its subsequent health effects. Some possible responses to the questions above might be:

1 The relationship between human activities, human health and sustainable development was outlined at the 1992 Rio Earth Summit (UN Conference on Environment and Development), where it was noted that human activities are compromised by ill health and degradation of the environment. For example, development cannot be sustained where water supplies are unsafe and where the waste products of human industry are allowed to pollute the environment.

2 Both infant and adult mortality are much higher in low-income than in high-income countries. There are a number of environmental factors that account for this difference, including a lack of safe water supplies and sanitation, overcrowding, squalid urban conditions and the inability to vaccinate against childhood illnesses. There will be more on these issues later in the book.

3 There is a difference between the sexes in the impact of the environment on health. Women are generally considered more vulnerable to environmental hazards because they are usually more directly involved with the basic living conditions – housing, sanitation and the provision of food and drinking water – on which these hazards have the biggest impact. This is covered more fully in later chapters on water, sanitation and air pollution.

Environment and health in your local area

Before moving on to examine environmental health in more depth in Chapter 2, it may be helpful to show the relevance of your studies to your everyday life. This activity requires you to think about the local area in which *you* live or work.

Activity 1.2

1 Find or draw a map of your local area – this could be your neighbourhood or village, and will require a scale with some level of detail. Go

for a 30-minute walk and mark up on the map any aspects of the outdoor environment that you consider important for health.

2   In this book we consider both the built and the natural environments. Make notes on the physical, biological and social hazards in the environment (use separate headings) that may affect human health.

Feedback

1   Your map could include the location of:
*   water pipes;
*   sewage works;
*   street drains;
*   locations where food is sold;
*   traffic areas – roads;
*   public transport – bus and train stations;
*   residential areas, including different housing types;
*   animal housing such as kennels or stables;
*   factories and industrial areas;
*   agricultural areas;
*   parks and other green spaces;
*   schools;
*   health services;
*   places of worship;
*   community centres.

2   Hazards you might have identified on the map of your area.

Physical and chemical hazards

*   Air pollution from roads and industrial areas/factories.
*   Road traffic collisions from road transport.
*   Flooding from the river.
*   Water pollution from industrial areas and from agriculture.

Biological hazards

*   Animals which are harmful to human health because they carry disease. For example, mosquitoes that carry malaria and breed in standing water. Animals that are kept near to human dwellings, with the potential to spread infectious disease.
*   Plant species which may produce pollen and other allergens.
*   Water pollution from abattoirs or farms (animal faeces).
*   Water pollution from sewage treatment works – depending on the level of treatment.

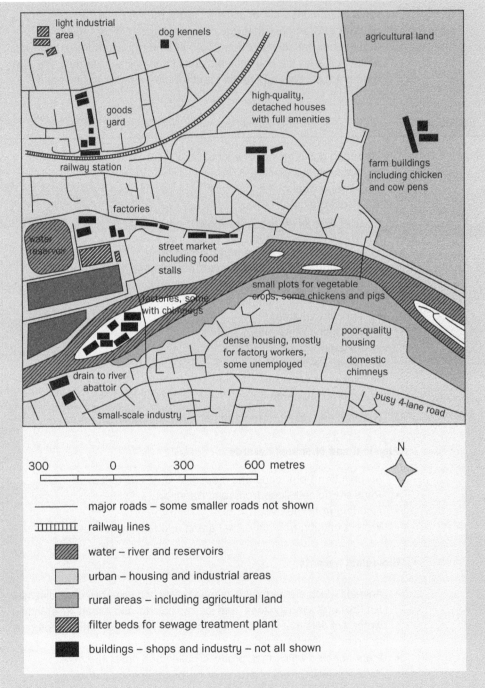

Figure 1.3 Environmental features of 'Ordinaryville'.

Social

- These factors are likely to be connected with poverty and social capital, for example, inadequate housing stock, lack of infrastructure (shops, roads, emergency services, utilities), social isolation and the effects of unemployment.

Built environment

- Some of the housing is of poor quality – this could exacerbate the spread of infectious diseases.
- Some of the roads are very busy, leading to possible problems with air pollution and traffic accidents.

Natural environment

- Parks and green spaces that benefit mental health and wellbeing.
- Local food production.

Some of the potential environmental problems depend on the quality of, and adherence to, local regulations concerning the housing of animals, food storage and service and industrial processes.

Summary

This chapter introduced definitions of health, environment and environmental health, and discussed the concept of sustainable development as used in this book. It has also shown that the environment plays a crucial role in human health and that it can both benefit and harm health: poor environmental quality is related to a significant burden of disease globally. The importance of sustainable development and its relationship to health and environmental quality have been introduced, along with approaches to its implementation. The cornerstone of sustainable development is the belief that everyone in the community should have access to a safe environment for health – and this includes future generations. The concept of environmental justice has been introduced, along with the potential for environmental effects to have a greater impact on vulnerable groups. If economic development does not meet the criteria for sustainability, this can lead to environmental damage, loss of biodiversity (with eventual disruption to global systems), damage to human systems and lack of equity in societies across both space (intra-generational equity) and time (inter-generational equity).

References

Frumkin, H. (ed.) (2010) *Environmental Health: from global to local*. San Francisco: Jossey-Bass.

HM Government (2005) *Securing the Future: Delivering UK Sustainable Development Strategy*, http://www.who.int/quantifying_ehimpacts/publications/ebddeaths2004corr.pdf, accessed 3 October 2012.

IISD (International Institute for Sustainable Development) (2012) http://www.iisd.org/about/, accessed 9 October 2012.

Kemp, R. and Parto, S. (2005) Governance for sustainable development: moving from theory to practice, *International Journal of Sustainable Development*, 8(1/2): 12–30.

Lehtonen, M. (2004) The environmental-social interface of sustainable development: capabilities, social capital, institutions, *Ecological Economics*, 49: 199–214.

Spangenberg, J.H. and Giljum, S. (2005) Editorial, *International Journal of Sustainable Development*, 8(1/2): 1–2.

SDC (Sustainable Development Commission) (2010) *Sustainable Development: the key to tackling health inequalities*. London: Sustainable Development Commission.

SDC (Sustainable Development Commission) (2011) What is sustainable development? http://www.sd-commission.org.uk/pages/what-is-sustainable-development.html, accessed 23 April 2014.

UCLG (United Cities and Local Governments) (2010) Culture 21: agenda for culture, http://www.agenda21culture.net/index.php, accessed 8 October 2012.

UNCED (1992) United Nations Conference on Environment and Development (UNCED), Rio de Janeiro, http://www.un.org/esa/sustdev/documents/UNCED_Docs.htm.

United Nations (1948) *Universal Declaration of Human Rights*. New York: UN.

United Nations (1993) *Earth Summit – Agenda 21*. New York: UN.

UNSCD (2012) UN Conference on Sustainable Development: the future we want, http://www.uncsd2012.org/content/documents/727The%20Future%20We%20Want%2019%20June%201230pm.pdf, accessed 29 April 2014.

WHO (1948) WHO definition of health, http://www.who.int/about/definition/en/, accessed 20 August 2004.

WHO (1986) *The Ottawa Charter for Health Promotion*. Geneva: WHO.

WHO (1987) *Our Common Future. Report to United Nations General Assembly* (A/RES/42/187), 11 December (the Brundtland report). Geneva: WHO.

WHO (1992) *Our Planet, Our Health*. Geneva: WHO.

WHO (1993) *Global Strategy: health, environment and development: approaches to drafting country-wide strategies for human well-being under Agenda 21*. Geneva: WHO.

WHO (2006) *Preventing Disease Through Healthy Environments: towards an estimate of the environmental burden of disease* (Prüss-Üstün, A. and Corvalán, C.), http://www.who.int/quantifying_ehimpacts/publications/preventingdisease.pdf, accessed 25 September 2015.

WHO (2010) *The Ottawa Charter for Health Promotion*, http://www.int/healthpromotion/conferences/previous/ottawa/, accessed 8 December 2010.

WHO (2016) Health impact assessment, glossary of terms used, http://www.who.int/hia/about/glos/en/index1.html, accessed 16 January 2016.

Assessing the impact of the environment on health

2

Emma Hutchinson and Sari Kovats

Overview

In this chapter, you will look at how the environment affects human health. Humans are exposed to different sources of environmental hazards, which may occur simultaneously or in isolation. Environmental hazards may be natural or result from human activities. Scientific evidence may be used to assess the impact of exposures on human health and to quantify the benefits of policies or strategies to reduce the exposures. You will be introduced to the requirements for a healthy environment and the importance of environmental justice. You will learn how health evidence can be used in environmental decision-making and look at frameworks and methods for quantifying the burden of disease due to environmental factors.

Learning objectives

By the end of this chapter you will be able to:

- understand the types of environmental hazard and how they affect health
- describe the basic requirements for a healthy environment and understand the importance of healthy settings
- apply frameworks used to describe complex environmental causes of health effects
- assess the role of health evidence in environmental decision-making

Key terms

Environmental exposure: The process by which an agent (from the environment) comes into contact with a person in such a way that the person may develop related outcomes, such as disease.

Environmental justice: The fair distribution of environmental benefits and burdens.

Externalities: Social benefits and costs that are not included in the market price of an economic good (Last 2001).

Hazard: A factor or exposure that may adversely affect health.

Health impact assessment (HIA): A means of assessing the health impacts of policies, plans and projects in diverse economic sectors using quantitative, qualitative and participatory techniques.

Inter-sectoral action for health: The promotion of health through the involvement of actors in other sectors, such as transport, housing and environmental regulation.

Precautionary principle: A principle that advocates the use of prudent social policy in the absence of comprehensive empirical evidence in an attempt to solve a problem. It enables a rapid response in the face of a possible danger to human, animal or plant health, or to protect the environment. In particular, where scientific data does not permit a complete evaluation of the risk, recourse to this principle may, for example, be used to stop the distribution or order withdrawal from the market of products likely to be hazardous (EU definition, from EUR-lex 2011).

Risk: The probability that an event will occur (Last 1995).

Risk assessment: The qualitative or quantitative estimation of the likelihood of adverse effects that may result from exposure to specified health hazards or from the absence of beneficial influences upon a target individual, group or population (Last 2001).

Health and the environment – introduction

The impact of humans on the environment

Biological, chemical and physical hazards have been in the environment throughout our history. Environmental hazards can be natural or of anthropogenic (human activity) origin. For example, arsenic is a naturally occurring contaminant of groundwater (see Chapter 4), whereas road transport is an anthropogenic cause of air pollution.

Unlike other species, humans have the ability to shape and control their environment, rather than be shaped by it. Some changes to the environment have been beneficial for health and wellbeing, such as improved housing and increased food production and water supply; but others are harmful, such as air and water pollution. Industrial pollution is not a new problem – even in ancient times, sites of production and manufacture were contaminated by pollutants. For example, lead contamination is still found in proximity to Roman metal smelters. When the scale of industry was small, the risks affected only the local environment and inhabitants. However, the environmental damage associated with modern industry is more widespread. The human influence on the environment is now so great that it has been argued we should rename the current geological time period the 'Anthropocene' (Zalasiewicz et al. 2010). This chapter discusses the impact of environmental hazards on health and introduces you to methods for assessing their impact. The changing pressures on the global environment are discussed in more detail in the next chapter (Chapter 3).

Box 2.1: The rise of environmental awareness

In the nineteenth century, awareness of the importance of the environment was increasing. By 1860, both the USA and UK had passed laws aimed at protecting the environment. Early environmental movements tended to be led by professionals such as foresters, who were interested in either the preservation or management of land and resources, such as the Sierra Club, an environmental organization in the USA founded in 1892. One of the first conservation campaigns in the USA was to protect Yosemite National Park, on the rationale that, 'Everybody needs beauty as well as bread, places to play in and pray in, where nature may heal and give strength to body and soul alike' (Muir 1912).

As the twentieth century progressed, there were rapid changes in the technologies associated with industrial development. At the same time, a growth in consumer demand led to huge increases in the volume of materials produced, and in the resultant pollution. Concern for the environment became more fragmented – the focus of public health had shifted to 'lifestyle' issues such as diet and exercise, rather than the environment. This trend continued until increasing levels of industrial pollution caused a massive public outcry in the 1960s and the 1970s in many parts of the world.

In her book *The Silent Spring* (1962), Rachel Carson detailed some of the dangers from large-scale use of pesticides. The book heightened public awareness of the pervasive and persistent nature of chemicals in the natural environment. At the same time, there was increasing concern over the effects of testing atomic weapons and the long-term contamination of the environment by radioactivity. Some major environmental disasters occurred, such as the grounding of the tanker *Torrey Canyon* which spilled 35 million gallons of crude oil off the coast of England in 1967.

These events were associated with a swelling of the membership of organizations concerned with environmental issues, and the birth of many new environmental organizations such as Greenpeace.

Paradigms for public health

The connections between health and the environment have been understood for a long time. However, the role of the environment as a determinant of health has been framed differently in different countries, and over different periods of time. It is useful for our understanding of developments in environmental health to consider how the approach to public health has changed over time. In high-income countries the first major changes occurred in the nineteenth century, with a focus on improving access to water and sanitation (Ashton 1991). These changes have also sometimes taken place in low- and middle-income countries (LMICs), but at different times in their histories. Overall, changes in public health thought and practice can be divided into six major time periods:

1 Public health as health protection, mediated though societies' social structures (antiquity–1830s).
2 The shaping of a distinct public health discipline by the sanitary movement ('miasma control', 1840s–70s).
3 Public health as contagion control (1880s–1930s).
4 Public health as preventive medicine (1940s–60s).
5 Public health as primary health care (1970s–80s).
6 Public health as health promotion (1990s–present).

A useful model for public health research is to consider the wide range of determinants of health, as shown in Figure 2.1. The main determinants of health can be described by individual factors (age, sex, genetic factors) and also the local environment (the built environment and the natural environment) (Dalhgren and Whitehead 1991). This model has been modified to take into account the importance of the global environment and ecosystem services (Barton and Grant 2006). For further discussion of public health methods see Sim and McKee (2011). In current public health practice, particularly in high-income countries, the focus has been on the social determinants of health (such as diet, physical activity, socioeconomic status, etc.), rather than the environmental determinants of health.

More recently, a new approach has been proposed (ecological public health) that integrates the social and environmental determinants of health. Rayner and Lang (2012) argue that public health should recognize the importance of the relationship between people, their circumstances and the biological world of nature and bodies. To put this concept in context, see the five models of public health presented in Table 2.1. These can be broadly mapped onto the six historical approaches listed above. It is important to consider how the core idea of how environment affects health has changed over time.

Finally, it is important to note that public health has always had a political dimension (McKee et al. 2011a). Public health is defined as the collective actions of society to benefit the health of populations. This assumes that

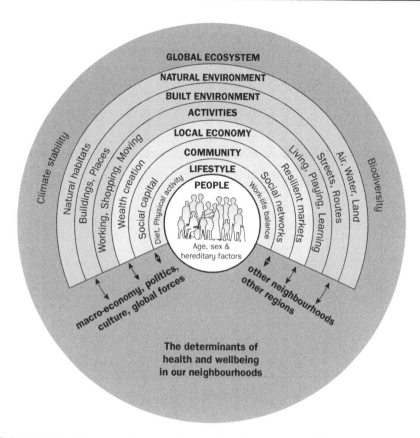

Figure 2.1 The main determinants of health: modified Dahlgren and Whitehead model of public health.

Source: Barton and Grant (2006) in Orme and Dooris (2010).

society exists (rather than a collection of individuals) and that society has responsibilities. Public health actions may also constrain the freedom of individuals in order to benefit the health of the population as a whole.

Environmental quality and health

Having considered the changing focus on environment in public health practice over time, we will now look at types of environmental hazard that affect human health and the different routes of exposure.

Environmental hazards

We depend on the environment for life. Maintaining and recycling resources obtained from the natural environment are essential for the supply of safe

Table 2.1 Five models of public health

	Sanitary environmental model	Social-behavioural model	Biomedical model	Techno-economic model	Ecological public health model
Core idea	The environment is a threat to health	Health is a function of knowledge and behaviour patterns	Health improvements require understanding of biological causation	Economic and technological growth is the prime elevator of health	Health depends on successful co-existence with the natural world and social relationships
Key methods	Engineering, product quality and regulation, licensing	Information campaigns, health literacy, social marketing	Two strands: individual medical interventions, population interventions	Scientific and product development, knowledge dissemination	Systems analysis in order to manage social transitions and create healthy habitats
Role of the state	Provision of services, funding, standards, town planning	Patron, educator, protector	Professional accreditation, formalization of education, medical support	Facilitator of economic growth, legislation, infrastructure	Coordination of action across sector/actors, protection of ecosystems
Main criticisms	Leaves out individuals; limited impact on modern lifestyle diseases	State interference reduces health to cognitive factors, underplays cultural determinants	Cost, reactive not proactive; narrow disciplinary base and concepts of prevention	Perverse impacts of economic growth	Too long term, requires system change; hard to initiate, downplays individual room for manoeuvre

Source: Modified from Rayner and Lang (2012)

food, drinking water and shelter. As individuals and populations consume more resources, increasing demands are placed on the environment.

Figure 2.2 illustrates the main categories of environmental hazards that affect health. Human activities such as transport, energy use, industry and agriculture, and urbanization determine the level of pollutants in the environment. Given the broad range of sectors giving rise to environmental hazards, addressing these hazards and the promotion of health requires the involvement of actors in other (non-health) sectors, such as transport, housing, etc. (Lock et al. 2011). Inter-sectoral collaboration for health is discussed in more detail in the topic-specific Chapters 4 to 9. Current approaches to public health also consider the physical and social aspects of people's surroundings – where they live, their local community, their home, and where they work and play (WHO 2010). Some of these aspects are developed further in Chapters 9 and 14. The idea of supportive environments is also developed later in this chapter, in the section on basic requirements for a healthy environment.

There are five main categories for the nature of hazard (see Figure 2.2). These are: biological (e.g. bacteria, viruses, parasites, other pathogenic organisms); chemical (e.g., toxic metals, air pollutants, solvents, pesticides); physical (e.g., radiation, temperature, noise); mechanical (e.g., traffic accidents, workplace injury); and social (e.g. stress, workplace discrimination, unemployment).

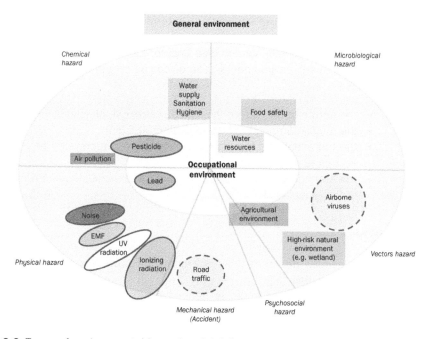

Figure 2.2 Types of environmental hazard and risk factors.
Source: WHO (2003).

Another way to categorize hazards is to consider the mechanisms by which humans come into contact with them (exposure route). The media that carry hazards include:

- water (used for drinking, recreational activities or agricultural activities such as irrigation);
- air (indoor and outdoor pollution);
- soil (also through consumption of food grown in contaminated soil);
- food (chemical and biological contamination);
- special environments that potentially carry hazards, such as agricultural environments, water resources or wetlands.

When we consider exposure routes, we need to think about how, to what, when and where we have been exposed. Therefore, we need to consider *how* we have been exposed – whether the exposure is by air, water, soil, etc.; *what* we may have been exposed to (a single exposure, multiple exposures); *when* we have been exposed (now, in the past, as a child, etc.) and *where* we have been exposed (home, work, school, community, hospitals).

You will read about environmental hazards, including air pollution, transport, water, chemical pollution, waste, disasters and energy production in more detail in later chapters. However, the environment should not just be seen as a source of specific health hazards. A more holistic approach can be developed in which the complex nature of the interaction between hazards is acknowledged. New types of hazard are manifesting at the global scale and which have implications in terms of local environmental effects – for example, damage to ecosystem services (see Chapter 13) and changes to the global climate system (see Chapter 12).

In summary, environmental hazards can be categorized in several different ways:

- the nature of the hazard (biological, chemical, physical);
- the media carrying the hazard (water, air, soil);
- the individual risk factors (e.g. living in an overcrowded house, lack of access to sanitation);
- the setting (e.g. the local environment, the occupational environment or at the global scale).

Hazards and risks

This section describes how environmental hazards can become risks to human health.

A *hazard*, in this book, is defined as 'a factor or exposure that may adversely affect health' (Last 2001). It is a qualitative term used to express the potential of an environmental agent to harm particular individuals if the exposure is above a certain level. An example of a hazard might be pesticide 'X' sprayed on apples.

A *risk* is defined as 'the probability that an event will occur, e.g. that an individual will become ill or die within a stated period of time or age; the probability of a (generally) unfavourable outcome' (Last 1995). In other words, a risk is the quantitative probability that a health effect will occur after an individual has been exposed to a specified amount of hazard. An example of a risk is the chance of developing cancer of the stomach after eating two apples a day for life (the exposure) which have been sprayed with pesticide 'X' (the hazard). A hazard only results in a risk if there has been an exposure – not if the hazard is contained or there is no opportunity for exposure. (Other slightly different definitions of risk exist, but the one we give here is that most current in public health.)

While we tend to concentrate on the health effects of single routes of exposure such as air pollution or waste disposal, in reality we are exposed to a cumulative number of environmental hazards, all of which impact upon our health. It is therefore a challenge to recognize the variety of exposures and act to mitigate these. For example, exposure to indoor air pollution, particularly in LMICs, has a significant adverse impact on health; however, there are also other hazards in the domestic environment, such as contaminated water, poor waste disposal and over-/under-insulation, leading to houses that are too cold or too hot. It is often important to consider the effect of all of these exposures on health, not just one in isolation.

✎ Activity 2.1

You have read about the range of environmental hazards that humans are exposed to. Table 2.2 details specific health conditions and specific environmental exposures – tick those boxes where you believe an association exists between the exposure and the health condition.

Table 2.2 Associations between environmental exposure and specific health outcomes

Health condition	Polluted air	Excreta and household waste	Polluted water or deficiencies in water management	Polluted food	Unhealthy housing
Acute respiratory disease	✓				✓
Diarrhoeal disease					
Malaria					
Poisonings					
Mental health conditions					
Cardiopulmonary diseases					
Cancer					
Chronic respiratory disease					

Source: Adapted from WHO (1997)

Feedback

Human health is clearly associated with exposure to a variety of hazards which need to be taken into account when developing health policies. For example, concentrating resources on tackling unhealthy housing will be associated with a positive impact on a range of health conditions including respiratory disease, injuries, cardiovascular disease, cancer and mental illness. If diarrhoea is to be tackled effectively, then policies relating to polluted food and water *as well as* sanitation need to be developed.

Some diseases are associated with a range of environmental exposures – acute respiratory disease, for instance, is associated with poor housing, overcrowding and indoor air pollution from biomass burning. This means that a range of solutions are required to reduce the burden of acute respiratory infection. Quantifying the burden of disease associated with different causes (exposures) can help target measures that will provide the biggest benefit in terms of deaths or cases avoided. Table 2.3 gives examples of some associations between various exposures and possible health outcomes.

Table 2.3 Associations between exposure and health outcomes

Health condition	Polluted air	Excreta and household waste	Polluted water or deficiencies in water management	Polluted food	Unhealthy housing
Acute respiratory disease	✓				✓
Diarrhoeal disease		✓	✓	✓	✓
Malaria		✓	✓		✓
Poisonings			✓	✓	✓
Mental health conditions					✓
Cardiopulmonary diseases	✓				
Cancer	✓			✓	
Chronic respiratory disease	✓				✓

Environmental risk transition

As countries undergo economic development, there are associated changes in potential environmental hazards which can lead to new health risks in the absence of sound environmental management (see Chapter 3; Smith and Ezzati 2005). This change in risk profile is referred to as the 'risk transition', and is further defined in this book as the process by which societies move from exposure to traditional hazards to exposure to modern hazards. Traditional hazards such as lack of access to water of sufficient quality or quantity, or lack of adequate food supply are still present in LMICs, while modern hazards such as lack of exercise, high fat diet and high levels of road traffic become more prevalent with increasing economic growth and specifically with increasing urbanization and industrialization, and the move away from agricultural to technology based economies.

✎ Activity 2.2

There are many types of environmental health hazard; these may vary according to a country's or an area's state of development. Read the following extract about Delhi, India. Make a list of traditional and a list of modern environmental hazards that you expect to affect health in this population.

Developmental activities in various sectors over the last decade resulted in huge migration. This influx of people has increased greatly in recent times putting the city under tremendous pressure of various kinds of pollution. The rapid growth of Delhi has resulted in significant increase in environmental pollution, such as air pollution, water pollution, noise pollution and also the pollution due to the municipal solid waste, bio-medical waste and hazardous waste etc. Ever increasing population in Delhi has resulted in various problems of cleaning up and disposal of waste generated in the city.

(Government of Delhi 2013)

Feedback

Table 2.4 describes some of the hazards you might have considered.

Table 2.4 Examples of traditional and modern health hazards in Delhi, India

Traditional hazards	Modern hazards
Lack of access to safe drinking water	Water pollution from populated areas or intensive agriculture
Inadequate or poor quality housing and shelter	
Inadequate basic sanitation (household and community)	Urban air pollution from motor cars, coal
Food contamination with pathogens, dietary deficiency	Food contamination with pesticides; poor diet leading to obesity

Indoor air pollution from cooking and heating using biomass fuel (wood, animal dung and crop residues)	Tobacco smoke
	Power stations and industry; traffic accidents
Disease vectors (mainly insects and rodents)	Emerging and re-emerging infectious disease hazards
Infectious agents	
Inadequate solid waste disposal	Solid and hazardous waste accumulation
Hazards of childbirth	
Occupational injury hazards in agriculture and cottage industries	Occupational injury from industry (e.g. large-scale machinery)
Wildlife and domestic animals	Chemical and radiation hazards from introduction of new technologies
Natural disasters, including floods, droughts and earthquakes	

Basic requirements for a healthy environment

In this section we will consider what the basic requirements for a healthy environment might be. This creates a starting point for policy-making at a local, national and global level that aims to ensure equity for all.

Healthy settings

The basic requirements for healthy environments form the basis for developing healthy settings. These are based on the concept of supportive environments, where people are called upon to actively engage in making environments more supportive to health (WHO 2010). This involves physical, social, spiritual, economic and political dimensions of people's environments. Four main aspects of supportive environments have been suggested: social, political, economic and the empowerment of women. Supportive environments encompass such aspects as good social networks, democratic participation in decision-making, and sustainable economic development – including transfer of technology, the greater participation of women and recognition of their skills and knowledge. All these aspects are believed to contribute towards a healthy and just society (WHO 2010).

Current thinking on supportive environments has led to policy approaches such as the healthy settings approach. The objective is to maximize disease prevention via a 'whole system' approach. The settings approach developed out of the WHO 'Health for All' strategy and, more specifically, the Ottawa Charter for Health Promotion (WHO 2012a, 2012b). According to the Ottawa Charter of 1986, 'Health is created and lived by people within the settings of their everyday life; where they learn, work, play, and love'.

Activity 2.3

Write down a list of aspects of the environment that you think are basic requirements for health.

Feedback

Understanding what constitutes a good environment for health helps us to make changes and improve health. The list below is not exhaustive:

- clean air;
- safe and sufficient water;
- adequate shelter – healthy housing, which gives protection from temperature extremes, damp, falls, and has safe water and sanitation;
- adequate and safe nutritious food;
- safe and peaceful settlements;
- access to education or employment;
- access to health care;
- security (free from conflict, violence and crime);
- protection from natural and technological hazards or disasters, such as flooding, landslides, earthquakes.

As such, healthy settings can be healthy cities, healthy workplaces, healthy schools, healthy homes, etc. There will be more discussion on the requirements for healthy housing in Chapter 6 and for healthy urban environments in Chapter 9.

Health in environmental decision-making

Having considered the ways in which environmental hazards can affect health, we now look at how to address these hazards. Here, and generally in the rest of this book, we will focus on the physical aspects of environment, the traditional area of environmental health. Environmental concerns relate to a range of hazards such as pesticides in food, contaminants in drinking water and toxic pollutants in the air. How do we determine which potential hazards really deserve attention? How do we, as a society, decide where to focus our efforts and resources to control these hazards?

Health risk assessment is a scientific tool designed to help answer these questions. It involves quantifying the burden of disease due to an environmental hazard. Government agencies rely on risk assessments to help them determine which potential hazards are the most significant. Risk assessments can also guide regulators in abating environmental hazards.

The DPSEEA framework was developed by the WHO to understand the linkages between environment and health, to support decision-making. The framework has been widely used in European and international health assessments (Corvalán et al. 2000). Figure 2.3 shows the framework. The range of causes that should be specified include the more immediate causes (exposures to environmental hazards) to more upstream causes of environmental hazards (such as environmental pressures caused by, e.g., economic or population growth). The immediate causes are termed *proximal* and the upstream causes *distal*.

* *Driving forces* or 'drivers' are the social, demographic and economic developments in societies (e.g., economic growth, urbanization) and the corresponding changes in lifestyle factors, overall levels of consumption and production patterns. Drivers function through human activities which may intentionally or unintentionally exert pressures on the environment.
* The *pressures* exerted by society may lead to unintentional or intentional changes in the *state* of the environment, such as levels of pollution in the water, air or soil.
* Factors such as human behaviour and lifestyle choice will influence individual *exposure* to environmental hazards. These exposures lead to *effects* on human health which include mortality and morbidity outcomes.
* *Action* can be taken by decision-makers at any stage along this causal chain.

An illustration of the DPSEEA framework as applied to a) outdoor air pollution and b) indoor air pollution is given in Table 2.5.

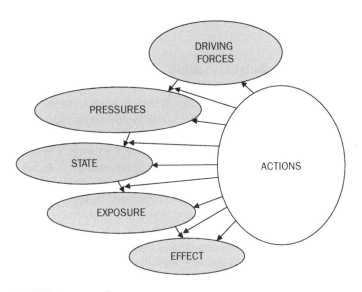

Figure 2.3 The DPSEEA framework.

Table 2.5 Application of the DPSEEA framework to air pollution

	Indoor air pollution	*Outdoor air pollution*
Driving forces	Energy policy, lack of access to clean energy, poverty	Transport policy, urban development, increased social demand for cars
Pressures	Emissions from household fuel use	Emissions from traffic, industry and power generation
State	Indoor air pollution	Outdoor air pollution
Exposures	Small particles, carbon monoxide	Particulate matter, carbon monoxide, ozone, nitrogen dioxide and sulphur dioxide
Effects	Acute lower respiratory infection (ALRI) in children, chronic obstuctive pulmonary disease (COPD) and lung cancer in adults, especially in women; risk of violence to women when fuel-gathering	Respiratory and cardiovascular mortality in adults; lung cancer
Action (based on general knowledge)	More efficient and less polluting cooking stoves; access to clean energy	Transport policy, emission reduction (e.g. catalytic converters)

Environmental justice

In response to the increasing awareness that the impact of the environment on health is not equal among all sectors of the population, the concept of *environmental justice* has developed. The environmental justice movement began in the USA in 1982 when North Carolina selected the Shocco township (which has a predominantly non-white population with a high proportion below the poverty line) to host a hazardous waste landfill containing chemically contaminated soil. Historically, environmental discrimination has occurred with respect to waste disposal, manufacturing (location of 'dirty' industries) and energy production (Land Loss Prevention Project 2006–13).

Environmental justice focuses on the fair distribution of environmental benefits and burdens (distributive justice) and meaningful participation in decision-making processes (procedural justice). It represents a developing approach in which what constitutes truly healthy, liveable, sustainable and vital communities is central (Lee 2002). Effective action to redress inequitable distributions of environmental burdens (such as pollution, industrial facilities and crime) may need to focus beyond exposure and consider social, economic and cultural factors, as introduced in Chapter 1 (Lee 2005). Figure 2.4 shows the pathways by which exposure to environmental hazards for different groups can lead to health inequalities.

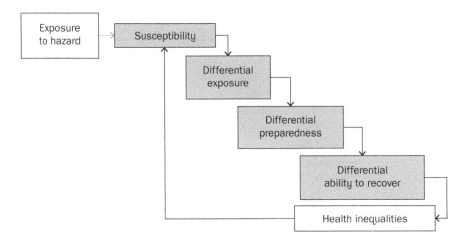

Figure 2.4 Environmental justice and health inequalities.

Source: Lee in Frumkin (2005).

Health inequalities (e.g. health status in lower income groups) may lead
to differences in susceptibility to environmental hazards (e.g. greater susceptibility to health effects associated with cold housing due to pre-existing
disease); differences in exposure (e.g. due to financial difficulties in providing adequate heating); differences in preparedness (e.g. lack of insulation);
and differences in ability to recover (e.g. inability to address a cold home
by supplying extra heating or applying energy efficiency measures). In this
case required action would need to focus on social and economic factors.
Other examples of this pathway include differential access to transportation, opportunities for walking and access to recreational facilities, depending on community factors (such as social cohesion and income) (Lee 2005).
Again, in this case, action on the wider determinants of health would be
required to address these issues. These could include cultural factors, such
as attitudes to walking and perception of crime.

Risk assessment

Risk assessment is the process of estimating risks to health attributable to
environmental hazards. It is defined as the qualitative or quantitative estimation of the likelihood of adverse effects that may result from exposure to
specified health hazards or from the absence of beneficial influences (Last
2001). Risk assessment uses clinical, toxicological, epidemiological, environmental and any other pertinent data. Risk assessment provides an estimate
of the health impacts of an environmental hazard or hazards, but the process
of risk characterization is used to communicate these impacts, and relies on
a combination of science and expert judgement, taking into account such

considerations as which and what type of communities would be affected (see the example of arsenic in drinking water discussed in Chapter 4).

Disease burden can be expressed in deaths, incidence or in disability-adjusted life years (DALYs) (see McKee et al. 2011b). The latter measure combines the burden due to death and disability in a single index. The DALY relies on an acceptance that the most appropriate measure of the effects of chronic illness is time, both time lost due to premature death and time spent disabled by disease. One DALY, therefore, is equal to one year of healthy life lost. Using such an index permits the comparison of the burden due to various environmental risk factors with other risk factors.

Economic considerations and externalities

Quantifying risks can help inform decision-makers about the costs and benefits of inaction on environmental policies. The health burdens (deaths, DALYs, lost activity days) are often converted to economic values in order to support decision-making using standard values. Thus health impacts can be considered as externalities when doing an economic analysis (or health impact assessment).

Externalities are social benefits and costs that are not included in the market price of an economic good (Last 2001). Individuals tend not to include the full environmental costs of activities in their decisions as to how much of a resource to 'consume'. When deciding, for example, how far to drive or how much coal to use to heat their homes, individuals tend only to consider the 'private' costs, such as fuel, and do not consider costs external to themselves (e.g. of polluting the atmosphere). Public goods such as clean air are not traded on markets and therefore do not have market prices. This is because they belong to everybody and nobody – there is a lack of clearly defined property rights and it is not possible to prevent someone from consuming them if they do not pay for them. In the absence of regulation, none of this pollution damage is paid for by the consumer, instead it is paid for by society in terms of ill health and environmental degradation. This can be addressed by policy interventions such as the 'polluter pays' principle – in which the marginal social cost (marginal private cost + marginal external cost) is equal to the price, and can be achieved by the use of such economic policy instruments as pollution taxes or tradeable permits.

Action to protect health from environmental hazards

Managing environmental risks requires us to develop the most appropriate strategies, policies or measures in response to an environmental hazard, taking into account all regulatory, political, environmental, engineering and social factors which might be relevant.

Historically, action to protect the environment has focused on eliminating or reducing significant hazards. The DPSEEA framework discussed above shows that action to prevent environmental hazards can be taken at all levels of policy (see Figure 2.3). Upstream prevention is likely to be more effective in protecting health, but is often more difficult to do (see Chapter 7 for an example relating to transport and health).

Current understanding on managing environmental risks recognizes the additional value of this being in a context of positive physical environments which nurture better health and wellbeing.

> *Creating safe and positive neighbourhoods for health requires us to think, plan and deliver in new and more effective ways. For example, the Scottish government is formulating policy which shapes places which are 'nurturing of positive health, wellbeing and resilience and which are consistent with and promoting of healthy behaviour and healthier lives'. . . The contribution of the physical surroundings to the health (both physical and mental) of those living in our most deprived areas of society is significant. This is a view increasingly supported by the flow of evidence. Indications are that the environment in poorer neighbourhoods in the UK is generally no more toxic or infectious than that of more affluent communities. Frequently though, such places are untidy, damaged and lacking in amenity. These factors create neighbourhoods which are often alienating and even threatening. Implicitly this contributes to a cocktail of disadvantage inconsistent with health and wellbeing for adults and children.*
>
> (The Scottish Government 2008)

It is not always possible to have complete information on potential health risks, as obtaining information on health risks associated with environmental hazards can be complex. Ideally, policy decisions are based on comprehensive information on health risks, but in some cases decision-makers deem it prudent to take policy actions in the absence of complete information – this is known as the *precautionary principle* (Martuzzi and Tickner 2004), and is included in the 1992 Rio Declaration on Environment and Development. It is now widely accepted as applying in situations where there is threat of harm to human, animal or plant health, as well as in the original context of preventing environmental damage (HSE 2013).

Examples where the precautionary principle has been clearly applied include limiting mobile phone use in children in the UK and limiting the use or release of genetically modified organisms into the environment (at least in the European Union). There are also several examples where the precautionary principle has failed to be applied (EEA 2001). For example, the adverse health effects of asbestos were first discovered in the 1900s with published reports of asbestosis associated with occupational exposures (Gee and Greenberg 2001). The first cases of mesothelioma (cancer associated with asbestos exposures) were described in the 1940s and 1950s, and asbestos was strongly suspected as the cause. Yet, regulations and the adequate enforcement of regulations to restrict the use of asbestos were not applied until the 1970s. Application of the precautionary principle would have led to regulatory action before the evidence was considered definitive. Earlier action would have avoided a large burden of disease due to the contaminant.

It has been argued that the types of precautionary action should be multiple in nature and case-specific (Martuzzi and Tickner 2004), depending on:

- the nature of the risk, its level of uncertainty, magnitude and reversibility;
- who is exposed (e.g. disproportionately affected or highly vulnerable communities);
- issues of technological and economic feasibility, benefits, proportionality and non-discrimination;
- preventability of risk;
- social values.

Summary

Historically, societies have approached the relationship between environment and health in various ways. With the rise of the importance of public health organizations and growing environmental awareness came recognition of the impact that the environment has on human health. In this chapter we have looked at hazards in the environment that affect human health, and the ways that these hazards can be categorized. In recent years, the impacts on health from environmental hazards have been extended to encompass the impact on health from the wider environment, including social, economic, cultural and political factors. This has led to the development of the concept of healthy settings for health. Finally, we have seen how the complex nature of the interaction between environment and health can be illustrated with the use of frameworks, and discussed the role of scientific assessment in informing policy.

References

Ashton, J. (1991) Sanitarian becomes ecologist: the new environmental health, *British Medical Journal*, 302: 189–90.

Barton, H. and Grant, M. (2006) A health map for the local human habitat, *Journal of the Royal Society for the Promotion of Public Health*, 126(6): 252–61.

Carson, R.L. (1962) *The Silent Spring*. London: Hamish Hamilton.

Corvalán, C., Briggs, D. and Zielhuis, G. (2000) *Decision-making in Environmental Health: from evidence to action*. London: E & FN Spon.

Dalhgren, G. and Whitehead, M. (1991) *Policies and strategies to promote social equity in health* (mimeo). Stockholm: Institute for Future Studies.

EEA (2001) *Late Lessons from Early Warning: the precautionary principle*. Copenhagen: European Environment Agency.

EUR-lex (2011) The precautionary principle, http://eur-lex.europa.eu/legal-content/EN/TXT/?uri=URIS-ERV:l32042, accessed 28 September 2015.

Gee, D. and Greenberg, M. (2001) Asbestos: from 'magic' to malevolent mineral, in EEA, *Late Lessons from Early Warning: the precautionary principle*. Copenhagen: European Environment Agency.

Government of Delhi, India, Department of Pollution (2013) http://www.delhi.gov.in/wps/wcm/connect/ Environment/environment/rti_manuals/particulars+of+organization, accessed 12 February 2013.

HSE (2013) *United Kingdom Interdepartmental Liaison Group on Risk Assessment (UK-ILGRA), the precautionary principle: policy and application*, http://www.hse.gov.uk/aboutus/meetings/committees/ ilgra/pppa.htm, accessed 13 August 2014.

Land Loss Prevention Project (LLPP) (2006–13) *Environmental Justice*, http://www.landloss.org/environmentaljustice.php, accessed 4 February 2013.

Last, J. (1995) *Dictionary of Epidemiology*, 3rd edn. Oxford: Oxford University Press.

Last, J. (2001) *Dictionary of Epidemiology*, 4th edn. New York: Oxford University Press.

Lee, C. (2002) Environmental justice: building a unified vision of health and the environment, *Environmental Health Perspectives* 110 (suppl. 2): 141–4.

Lee, C. (2005) Environmental justice, in H. Frumkin (ed.) *Environmental Health: from global to local*. San Francisco: Jossey-Bass.

Lock, K. et al. (2011) Assessing the impact on population health policies in other sectors, in F. Sim and M. McKee (eds) *Issues in Public Health*, 2nd edn. Maidenhead: Open University Press.

Martuzzi, M. and Tickner, J.A. (eds) (2004) *The Precautionary Principle: protecting public health, the environment and the future of our children*. Copenhagen: WHO.

McKee, M., Sim, F. and Pomerleau, J. (2011a) The emergence of public health and the centrality of values, in F. Sim and M. McKee (eds) *Issues in Public Health*, 2nd edn. Maidenhead: Open University Press.

McKee, M. et al. (2011b) Understanding the burden of disease using the available data, in F. Sim and M. McKee (eds) *Issues in Public Health*, 2nd edn. Maidenhead: Open University Press.

Muir, J. (1912) *The Yosemite*. New York: The Century Co., http://vault.sierraclub.org/john_muir_exhibit/ writings/the_yosemite/, accessed 28 September 2015.

Orme, J. and Dooris, M. (2010) Integrating health and sustainability: the higher education sector as a timely catalyst, *Health Education Research*, 25(3): 425–37.

Rayner, G. and Lang, T. (2012) *Ecological Public Health: reshaping the conditions for good health*. London: Routledge.

Sim, F. and McKee, M. (eds) (2011) *Issues in Public Health, 2nd edn*. Maidenhead: Open University Press.

Smith, K.R. and Ezzati, M. (2005) How environmental risks change with development: the epidemiologic and environmental risk transitions revisited, *Annual Review of Environment and Resources*, 30: 291–333.

The Scottish Government (2008) *Good Places, Better Health*, www.scotland.gov.uk/Resource/Doc/254447/ 0075343.pdf.

WHO (1997) *Environment, Health and Sustainable Development*. Geneva: WHO.

WHO (2003) Assessing the environmental burden of disease at national and local levels, in A. Prüss-Üstün, D. Campbell-Lendrum, C. Corvalán and A. Woodward (eds) *Environmental Burden of Disease*, http://www. who.int/quantifying_ehimpacts/publications/en/9241546204.pdf, accessed 8 March 2016.

WHO (2010) *WHO Healthy Workplace Framework and Model: background and supporting literature and practices*, http://www.who.int/occupational_health/publications/healthy_workplaces_background_ documentdfinal.pdf, accessed 12 February 2013.

WHO (2012a) *Introduction to Health Settings*, http://www.who.int/healthy_settings/about/en/index. html, accessed 16 October 2012.

WHO (Collaborating Centre for Healthy Urban Environments) (2012b) *What is a Healthy Urban Environment?*, http://www.bne.uwe.ac.uk/who/what.asp, accessed 16 October 2012.

Zalasiewicz, J. et al. (2010) The new world of the Anthropocene, *Environmental Science & Technology*, 44(7): 2228–31.

Changing pressures on health and the environment 3

Sari Kovats and Emma Hutchinson

Overview

In this chapter, you will be introduced to the concepts of the demographic, epidemiological and urban transitions as populations experience rapid social and economic change. The causes of this rapid change (population growth, urbanization, technological development and increases in consumption) are also important drivers of resource depletion and environmental pollution. These are all aspects of global environmental change. In this chapter we will look at how these increasing pressures interact with the environment and the implications of this for public health.

Learning objectives

By the end of this chapter you will be able to:

- understand the implications of demographic, epidemiological and urban transitions for the health of populations
- describe the linkages between global environmental change and health

Key terms

Demographic transition: The transition from high to low fertility and high to low child mortality rates in a country.

Environmental risk transition: The changing pattern of environmental hazards that accompany economic development.

Epidemiological transition: Changing patterns of disease, from high burdens of infectious diseases and malnutrition to increased incidence of non-communicable diseases. It is closely associated with the demographic transition.

Global environmental change: Environmental changes that affect global earth systems, such as climate change.

Urban transition: Increasing proportion of a nation's population living in urban areas, also called 'urbanization'.

Introduction

In this chapter we discuss in more detail the 'upstream' factors that affect human health, also termed 'human driving forces' according to the DPSEEA framework described in Chapter 2 (WHO 1997).

Human activities such as economic growth, the provision and use of services and increasing household consumption are contributing to the global environmental changes that have implications for human health. In particular, resource depletion and environmental degradation are undermining the ecosystem services upon which human populations depend. (See Chapter 13 for further details on ecosystem services, which is a framework that describes how the natural environment benefits health and wellbeing by providing provisioning services – food and shelter – regulating services – cleaning the air and water – and cultural services – landscapes that people enjoy.) The adverse human and environmental consequences of such unsustainable development at a global scale include transboundary air pollution, deforestation, climate change and loss of biodiversity.

In terms of environmental impacts on health, it is not enough to understand how exposure to an isolated chemical air pollutant (e.g. PM_{10}) might affect an individual; we also need to know how and why the individual is exposed, including the upstream driving forces. As discussed in Activity 2.4 on outdoor air pollution, these driving forces include the urban transition, economic development and the type of transport and energy policies that are in place (as well as how well they are implemented). How governments legislate and create programmes to deal with these driving forces is important in mitigating (reducing) environmental threats to health. A detailed discussion on policy-making is outside the scope of this book, but some examples of local, national and international environmental policies relevant to environment and health are described in Chapter 14.

Much environment and health research is focused on the proximal types of hazard (immediate and local), such as air pollutants or chemicals in the water supply. Scientific methods and tools, such as epidemiology and risk assessment, are best able to quantify risks associated with these kinds of risk factors. McMichael (1998) has described epidemiologists as the 'prisoners of the proximate' because they focus on proximate factors as the causes of disease. While this type of research has been important in identifying and managing such risk factors, this chapter aims to describe some of the important 'distal' (upstream) determinants of population health.

Environmental risk transition

As a country undergoes economic development there are associated changes in exposures to environmental hazards which, in the absence of good environmental management, can lead to new health risks (Smith and Ezzati 2006). This is termed the 'environmental risk transition' and is defined in this book as the process by which individuals in a population move over time from exposure to traditional hazards to exposure to modern hazards. The term 'risk transition' has also been used to describe changes in a wide range of risk factors, not just environmental ones (McKee et al. 2011).

The risk transition concept is closely related to the 'epidemiological transition' which is the change in the distribution of diseases in a given population, with a decline in infectious diseases and an increase in incidence of non-communicable diseases, such as cancer, diabetes, and cardiovascular and respiratory disease. The reasons for this are outlined below.

The previous chapter discussed the categories of 'traditional' and 'modern' environmental risks (Activity 2.2). In a given country or population, economic development generally improves living standards, infrastructure and health service provision so that exposure to traditional hazards are reduced in the long term. However, rapid economic development together with a lack of regulation can lead to two things. First, it can impede the improvement in exposure to traditional environmental risks, such as from poor access to water and sanitation and poor access to

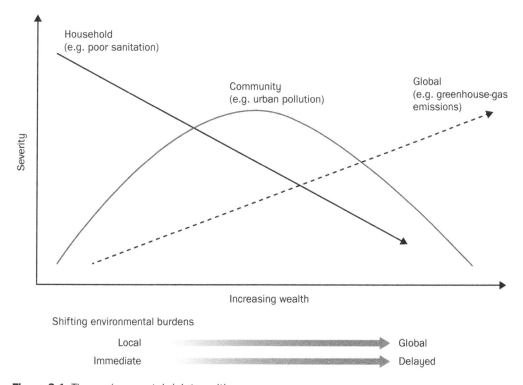

Figure 3.1 The environmental risk transition.

Source: Holdren and Smith (2000).

clean energy. Second, economic development has been associated with an increase in 'modern' environmental health risks, such as outdoor air pollution and chemical exposures from increased industrialization and modern agricultural practices, as well as traffic accidents from increasing use of road transport. These risks can increase before environmental management and other policies reduce the risks over time. This is shown in Figure 3.1.

 Activity 3.1

Consider your country. What are the most important environmental health hazards in your country now? What are the proximate and upstream (distal) causes? What have been the main changes in environmental health risks over the last 20 years?

Feedback

The environmental risks will differ, depending on where you live. You could look at the website of your National Ministry of Health or Ministry of Environment and see what environmental health problems are listed there. For example, common environmental concerns include outdoor air pollution and chemicals in the environment. These environmental hazards are considered 'proximate' as they are closely linked to direct exposures to individuals.

Upstream causes in low-income countries may be related to population growth, urbanization or even economic development, such as a shift from an agricultural-based economy to an industrialized economy.
The main changes in environmental health risks over the last 20 years in high-income countries may be related to air pollution and energy use. Some searching of your government's health and environmental websites may identify other specific changes in environmental health risks in your location.

Demographic transition

The world's population is growing and expected to peak in size at about the middle of this century (UNPD 2011). In 2011, the world's population reached 7 billion people; more than a doubling of the population over the past 40 years (UNPD 2011). Figure 3.2 shows that the majority of future projected increases in populations will occur in Africa and Asia.

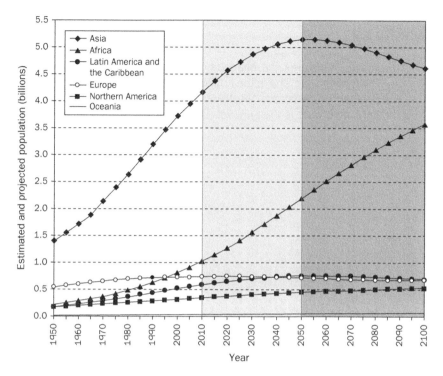

Figure 3.2 Estimated and projected population by major area, medium variant, 1950–2100 (billions).
Source: UNPD (2011).

Population dynamics have complex implications for public health, and three separate aspects need to be considered:

- population growth;
- population ageing;
- population movement (temporary or permanent migration).

The demographic transition is the change within a population from high birth rate and high child mortality to low birth rate and low child mortality. It entails a change in the population age structure from a high proportion of children before the demographic transition to a greater proportion of older people (the ageing population) thereafter.

The transition was formerly thought to be a consequence of technological change and industrialization, but it is also directly related to increasing female literacy and improvements in the status of women. It is estimated that in the early part of the twenty-first century approximately 20 million women in low- and middle-income countries (LMICs) are unable to access contraceptives or good quality family planning services, either because they are unavailable or because social and economic forces prevent them from taking advantage of these services even where they are available (UNFPA, 2012).

Activity 3.2

Figure 3.3 shows the changes in mortality patterns in a rural area of Bangladesh. How have the environmental risks changed over time in this population? What are the likely driving forces of these environmental risks, and what is their impact on mortality?

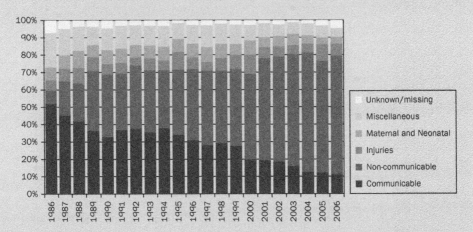

Figure 3.3 Changes in mortality by cause of death in rural Bangladesh, 1986–2006.
Source: Karar et al. (2009).

Feedback

1　There is steep decline in the proportion of deaths from infectious (communicable) diseases. This is accompanied by an increase in the proportion of deaths from non-communicable diseases. The proportion of deaths from injuries and maternal causes has stayed relatively stable over time.

2　Possible reasons for the decline in infectious diseases are likely to include: improvements in vector control; improved access to safe water and sanitation; increased immunization rates.

3　The increase in incidence of non-communicable diseases is likely to be related to changes in diet and lifestyle. Increases in cancer incidence may perhaps be associated with past increases in tobacco smoking. On the other hand, fewer indoor cook stoves (and replacement with the use of clean energy) will have reduced the burden of mortality from acute respiratory infections.

4　The likely upstream causes (driving forces) may include economic development leading to a change in diet, lower levels of physical activity and lifestyle factors including changes in smoking patterns and increased exposure to chemical hazards.

The urban transition

The 'urban transition' describes the shift in populations from rural to urban settings. This transition presents qualitatively new challenges for public health (Rayner and Lang 2012; WHO 2012a). The growth in urban populations has been very rapid, particularly in Asia. The United Nations projects that Africa's urban population will increase from 414 million to over 1.2 billion by 2050, while that of Asia will increase from 1.9 billion to 3.3 billion. The two regions together will account for 86 per cent of the increase in the world's urban population (UNPD 2012).

The concept of driving forces that influence health and the environment is particularly appropriate in the urban situation. The main driving force for urbanization is economic growth, particularly where manufacturing and services are the growth areas. Most large cities are in the world's largest economies. Economic growth is reflected in structural changes to a nation's economy; in growing economies the agricultural sector tends to decline, while the industry and services sectors (which are based in urban areas) tend to increase.

One of the potential consequences of population influx into cities is that it may occur at a faster rate than the infrastructural development can cope with. This situation may lead to a lack of adequate services, such as water supply and sanitation, lack of good quality housing and a corresponding increase in inequality between the newcomers and the established inhabitants of the city. Within a rapidly urbanizing area, particularly in low-income countries, social and economic conditions are often uncoordinated or, as McMichael (2000) puts it, 'Rapid urbanization represents a profound transformation . . . generally outstripping social and political responses'. Further discussion on the health impacts of rapid urbanization is given in Chapter 9.

Technological transitions

Along with the increase in population in the past 200 years, there have been considerable developments in our understanding of the world in which we live and our ability to control some aspects of it. Thus, science and technology have become significant influences on human health and the environment. Some economists tie population, consumption and technology together to describe their relative impacts on the environment, represented by the following equation (Chertow 2001):

$$I = PAT$$

$$(\text{impact} = \text{population} \times \text{affluence} \times \text{technology})$$

In high-income countries, scientific and technological developments have made significant contributions to the economy. Such developments have led to increased efficiency in agricultural and industrial production and improved health care, and increased access to education. However, these developments are not all positive, as they also allow the development of inefficient technologies and the production of pollutants and waste products (see Chapters 7 and 8). As populations grow and consumption increases, the use of technology to create greater efficiencies in energy production and industrial processes becomes increasingly important.

✎ Activity 3.3

Read this abstract, then briefly list the benefits and harms to public health associated with rapid economic development that are mediated through changes to the environment.

Environmental risk factors, especially air and water pollution, are a major source of morbidity and mortality in China. Biomass fuel and coal are burned for cooking and heating in almost all rural and many urban households, resulting in severe indoor air pollution that contributes greatly to the burden of disease. Many communities lack access to safe drinking water and sanitation, and thus the risk of waterborne disease in many regions is high. At the same time, China is rapidly industrialising with associated increases in energy use and industrial waste. Although economic growth from industrialisation has improved health and quality of life indicators, it has also increased the release of chemical toxins into the environment and the rate of environmental disasters, with severe effects on health. Air quality in China's cities is among the worst in the world, and industrial water pollution has become a widespread health hazard. Moreover, emissions of climate-warming greenhouse gases from energy use are rapidly increasing. Global climate change will inevitably intensify China's environmental health troubles, with potentially catastrophic outcomes from major shifts in temperature and precipitation. Facing the overlap of traditional, modern, and emerging environmental dilemmas, China has committed substantial resources to environmental improvement.

(Zhang et al. 2010)

Feedback

There are a range of impacts, both harmful and beneficial.

- Harmful health impacts of water and air pollution. Urban air pollution is a particularly serious problem in China, due to the rapid growth in manufacturing, use of motorized transport and lack of regulation.

- Longer-term impacts of degradation of the environment, particularly water and soil degradation which will have harmful implications for food production and, possibly, future food security.
- There will be potentially negative global impacts on health from greenhouse gas emissions.
- Benefits from economic development include improved income and lifestyles for much of the population. These are usually associated with increased life expectancy and a reduction in communicable diseases. However, this is often not equally distributed among the population as the next section will explain.

Trends in poverty and inequality

Although many countries have improved health outcomes at a population level, these improvements have not been shared equally by all people. The groups living in absolute poverty (sometimes measured as living on less than US$1 a day) are those who lack access to basic human requirements such as food, safe drinking water, sanitation facilities, health, shelter, education, employment and health care, and include a high proportion of women, children, refugees and other displaced persons (WHO 1996).

The WHO Commission on Social Determinants of Health recommended three principles of action (WHO 2012b):

1 Improve the conditions of daily life – the circumstances in which people are born, grow up, live, work and age.
2 Tackle the inequitable distribution of power, money and resources – the structural drivers of those conditions of daily life – globally, nationally and locally.
3 Measure the problem, evaluate action, expand the knowledge base, develop a workforce that is trained to address the social determinants of health, and raise awareness of the social determinants of health with the general public.

Inequalities are present in all countries. Table 3.1 lists actions that can be undertaken to improve population health where these inequalities exist and describes the evidence for each. Many of these inequalities are manifested through local environmental conditions such as access to secure housing, sanitation and clean water, and sufficient food of good quality.

These examples of actions are not always easy to implement, particularly where there is a lack of strong local government. Inequalities in health outcomes are associated with inequalities in the exposures to environmental hazards and these are discussed later in the book in topic-specific chapters.

Table 3.1 Examples of actions to reduce inequities in health in urban areas

Action	Evidence base
Improve daily living conditions	Good nutrition is crucial and begins *in utero* with adequately nourished mothers. Mothers and children need a continuum of care from pre-pregnancy, through pregnancy and childbirth, to the early days and years of life. Children need safe, healthy, supporting, nurturing, caring and responsive living environments.
Place health and health equity at the heart of urban governance and planning	Access to quality housing and shelter and clean water and sanitation are human rights and basic requirements for healthy living. The planning and design of urban environments has a major impact on health equity through its influence on behaviour and safety.
Establish and strengthen universal comprehensive social protection policies that support a level of income sufficient for healthy living for all	Low living standards are a powerful determinant of health inequity. They influence lifelong trajectories. Child poverty and transmission of poverty from generation to generation are major obstacles to improving population health and reducing health inequity.
Make full and fair employment and decent work a central goal of national and international social and economic policy-making	Work is the area where many of the important influences on health are played out. This includes both employment conditions and the nature of work itself. A flexible workforce is seen as good for economic competitiveness but brings with it negative effects on health. Poor mental health outcomes are associated with precarious employment. Workers who perceive work insecurity experience significant adverse effects on their physical and mental health.
Build health care systems based on principles of equity, disease prevention and health promotion	With partial health care systems, or systems with inequitable provision, opportunities for universal health as a matter of social justice are lost. These are core issues for all countries. More pressingly, for low-income countries, accessible and appropriately designed and managed health care systems will contribute significantly to the achievement of the Millennium Development Goals (MDGs), and will continue to contribute to their replacement, the Sustainable Development Goals (SDGs).

Source: WHO (2012b)

Globally, trends in poverty are declining. The MDG target of reducing extreme poverty rates by half was met five years ahead of the 2015 deadline. However, at the global level more than 800 million people are still living in extreme poverty (UN 2015).

Accelerating trends and the Earth system approach

The large-scale changes to the environment, such as urbanization and cutting down forests to convert the land to agricultural use, has allowed many benefits for human health. Such processes have reduced biodiversity but at the same time have provided food for the growing human population and improved living standards. Some have argued that these activities cannot continue indefinitely because they are causing irreversible damage to the world's ecosystems, to the extent that they will no longer function and provide those (ecosystem) services upon which humans depend (McMichael and Butler 2011). As environmentalism was emerging as a political movement in the 1970s, this pessimistic view was articulated in the book *Limits to Growth* (Meadows and Meadows 1972) which used modelling to project future trends of population growth, consumption, food production and environmental pollution. It discussed the implications of these projections in a world with finite resources. These concerns have been avoided, in the most part, by technological advances, particularly the 'Green Revolution' which greatly increased food productivity in the 1970s and 80s. However, concerns remain about the accelerating trends in consumption and resource use (Meadows et al. 2004).

The idea of global limits or 'tipping points' has been updated in the concept of planetary boundaries, proposed by Rockström et al. (2009). These planetary boundaries are irreversible changes in the Earth system which are likely to have serious adverse consequences for humanity including:

- climate change;
- ocean acidification;
- stratospheric ozone depletion;
- interference with the global phosphorus and nitrogen cycles;
- rate of biodiversity loss;
- global fresh water use;
- land system change;
- aerosol loading;
- chemical pollution.

Two boundaries were assessed as having already been exceeded: biodiversity loss and greenhouse gas emissions, which cause climate change. Some of these planetary boundaries are discussed in later chapters in this book: stratospheric ozone depletion and climate change (Chapter 12), biodiversity and land use change/deforestation (Chapter 13) and chemical pollution (Chapter 4). The evidence of the negative health effects of these large-scale changes is often used to justify international action to reduce their harmful effects (see Chapter 14).

Global environmental change and health

Global environmental changes are those that affect the Earth's system, either because the problems are so pervasive (e.g. biodiversity loss) or

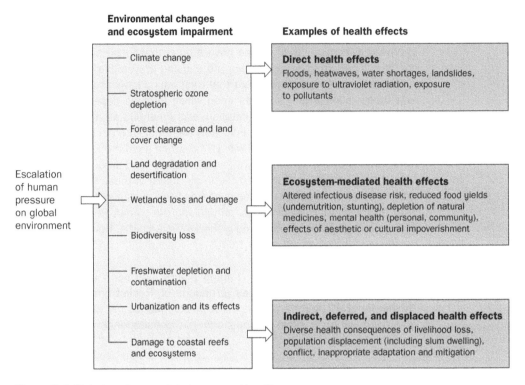

Figure 3.4 Global environmental change and health.
Source: Whitmee et al. (2015).

because a global system is being affected (e.g. changes in the climate system). Figure 3.4 illustrates the main types of global environmental change that are now of concern to human populations.

The scientific evidence that adverse global environment change will damage health in the future is accumulating. Environmental changes will undermine some of the scientific, technological and social progress which has led to the large increase in global life expectancy observed since 1950 (McMichael and Butler 2011). While local environmental risks still have significant impacts on human health, the biggest threat to global health appears to be from a cascade of future adverse environmental effects. Reducing this risk is vital not just for environmental integrity, but also to protect future population health. Much can be done to promote technologies, policies and strategies in order to improve the health of human populations and environmental conditions and this is discussed in Chapter 14.

Future directions for planet Earth and the Sustainable Development Goals

The MDGs were an international initiative to address the inequalities that affected the health of low-income populations. However, it has now been recognized that future development goals should address both reducing poverty and increasing environmental sustainability. The final target year for the MDGs was 2015 and they are now replaced by the SDGs (Sachs 2012). The SDGs apply to all countries (high-, middle- and low-income) which is an acknowledgment of the role all countries have to play in sustainable development. A critical analysis of the MDGs and recommendations arising from their challenges and successes is presented in Chapter 14 (see also Waage et al. 2010).

The SDGs build upon the MDGs and converge with the post-2015 development agenda (Waage et al. 2015). The goals on human wellbeing (which are central) are dependent on those that support infrastructure and the supporting natural systems. The proposed SDGs underscore the need for strong governance to ensure that infrastructure goals are not achieved at the expense of the supporting natural systems (Whitmee et al. 2015).

Summary

You will have seen the importance of human driving forces – such as demographic change, the urban transition, technology and economic development – in alleviating or exacerbating the effects of the environment on health. As discussed earlier, how societies move from traditional to modern hazards is known as the 'risk transition'. It can be argued that progress has been made in curtailing potential damage to the environment; however, much remains to be done, particularly as global economic development and natural resource use increase.

References

Chertow, M.R. (2001) The IPAT equation and its variants: changing views of technology and environmental impact, *Journal of Industrial Ecology*, 4(4): 13–29. http://mitpress.mit.edu/journals/pdf/jiec_4_4_13_0.pdf

Holdren, J.P. and Smith, K.R. (2000) Energy, the environment & health, in *World Energy Assessment: energy & the challenge of sustainability*. New York: UNDP/CSD/WEC.

Karar, A.Z., Alam, N. and Streatfield, K.P. (2009) Epidemiological transition in rural Bangladesh, 1986–2006, *Global Health Action*, 2, n. 2008.

McKee, M., Karanikolos, M., Sim, F. and Pomerleau, J. (2011) Understanding the burden of disease: using the available data, in F. Sim and M. McKee (eds) *Issues in Public Health, 2nd edn*. Maidenhead: Open University Press.

McMichael, A.J. (1998) Prisoners of the proximate: loosening the constraints on epidemiology in an age of change, *American Journal of Epidemiology*, 149(10): 887–97.

McMichael, A.J. (2000) The urban environment and health in a world of increasing globalization: issues for developing countries, *Bulletin of the World Health Organization*, 78(9).

McMichael, A.J. and Butler, C.D. (2011) Promoting global population health while constraining the environmental footprint, *Annual Review of Public Health*, 32: 179–97.

Meadows, D. and Meadows, D. (1972) *The Limits to Growth: a report for the Club of Rome's Project on the Predicament of Mankind*. Washington, DC: Potomac Associates.

Meadows, D., Randers, J. and Meadows, D.L. (2004) *Limits to Growth: the 30-year update*. Vermont: Chelsea Green Publishing.

Rayner, G. and Lang, T. (2012) *Ecological Public Health: reshaping the conditions for good health*. London: Routledge.

Rockström, J. et al. (2009) A safe operating space for humanity, *Nature*, 461: 472–5.

Sachs, J.D. (2012) From Millennium Goals to Sustainable Development Goals, *Lancet*, 379: 2206–11.

Smith, K.R. and Ezzati, M. (2006) How environmental health risks change with development: the epidemiologic and environmental risk transitions revisited, *Annual Review of Environment and Resources*, 30: 291–333.

UN (2015) www.un.org/millenniumgoals/poverty.shtml, accessed 2 October 2015.

UNFPA (2012) By choice, not by chance. Family planning, human rights and development, in *State of the World Population Report*. New York: UN Population Fund.

UNPD (2011) *World Population Prospects: the 2010 revision*. New York: United Nations Department of Economic and Social Affairs, Population Division.

UNPD (2012) *World Urbanization Prospects: the 2011 revision*. New York: United Nations Department of Economic and Social Affairs, Population Division.

Waage, J. et al. (2010). The Millennium Development Goals: a cross-sectoral analysis and principles for goal setting after 2015, *Lancet*, 376(9745): 991–1023.

Waage, J., Yap, C., Bell, S. et al. (2015) Governing the UN Sustainable Development Goals: interactions, infrastructure and institutions, *Lancet Global Health*, 3: e251–2.

Whitmee, S., Haines, A., Beyer, C. et al. (2015) Safeguarding human health in the Anthropocene epoch: report of The Rockefeller Foundation – *Lancet* Commission on Planetary Health. *Lancet*, Published July 2015.

WHO (1996) *World Health Report: fighting disease, fostering development*. Geneva: WHO.

WHO (1997) *Environment, Health and Sustainable Development*. Geneva: WHO.

WHO (2012a) *World Conference on Social Determinants of Health: meeting report*, Rio de Janeiro, Brazil, 19–21 October 2011. Generva: WHO.

WHO (2012b) *Closing the Gap in a Generation*. Geneva: WHO.

Zhang, J., Mauzerall, D.L., Zhu, T., Liang, S., Ezzati, M. and Remais, J.V. (2010) Environmental health in China: progress towards clean air and safe water, *Lancet*, 375(9720): 1110–9.

SECTION 2

Environmental hazards

Chemicals in the environment

Maria-Jose Lopez-Espinosa and Debapriya Mondal

4

Overview

Chemicals in the environment present a range of risks to human health. In this chapter, you will learn about the scientific methods used to identify sources of exposure, determine health effects and quantify health impacts. Three case studies of environmental chemicals are explored: arsenic, asbestos and persistent organic pollutants (POPs). Once a chemical has been assessed as posing a risk to human health, there are several policy options for risk management, including regulating the amount released into the environment.

Learning objectives

By the end of this chapter you will be able to:

- describe the range of contexts where chemicals in the environment impact on human health
- understand the various routes by which humans are exposed to chemicals in the environment
- describe the effects of selected chemicals on human health
- evaluate the methods used to estimate the impacts of environmental chemical exposures on human health
- evaluate policies, strategies and methods used to limit exposure to chemicals in the environment

Key terms

Bioaccumulation: Storage of a stable substance in living tissues, resulting in a much higher concentration than in the environment.

Biomagnification: Increase in the concentration of a substance through the food chain, i.e. from prey to predator (presupposes bioaccumulation).

Carcinogen: Cancer-causing agent.

Dose: A stated quantity or concentration of a substance to which an organism is exposed over either a continuous or an intermittent period.

Half-life of a chemical: The time required for a quantity of a substance to decay to half its concentration in the body or the environment as measured at the beginning of the time period.

Risk assessment: The qualitative or quantitative estimation of the likelihood of adverse effects that may result from exposure to specified health hazards or from the absence of beneficial influences upon a target individual, group or population. Risk assessment uses clinical, toxicological, epidemiological, environmental and any other pertinent data.

Risk management: The process of identification, analysis, assessment, control and avoidance, minimization or elimination of risks. Risk management uses risk assessment in combination with socioeconomic and political inputs to evaluate and select measures to manage risk.

Introduction

There are more than 10 million recognized chemicals in the world (EEA 2011). Many of them play a key role in the provision of the goods and services that support our lifestyles and economies. However, even small amounts of some of these chemicals can endanger human health. Some are discharged into the environment during natural processes (e.g. the release of arsenic into the ground water from minerals); others are discharged during mining, milling or manufacturing of products (e.g. asbestos). and others are man-made chemicals, which are found in pesticides, textiles, plastics and electrical goods (e.g., POPs).

Few of the large number of chemical substances manufactured have gone through any evaluation of their possible long-term human health effects. Concern about this in Europe led to the introduction of the REACH (Registration, Evaluation, Authorization and Restriction of Chemicals) Regulation in 2007. The objective of REACH is that industries themselves should ensure in advance that the chemicals they manufacture and put on the market in the European Union do not adversely affect human health or the environment. REACH applies to both new and existing chemicals. It is considered the strictest law to date regulating chemical substances in the world (European Commission 2007).

Environmental health risk assessment

Risk assessment, as introduced in Chapter 2, is one of the methods used to evaluate the potential for adverse health effects in humans from exposure to environmental hazards. Risk assessment, also known as health risk assessment or environmental health risk assessment, has four separate steps (NRC 1983):

1 *Hazard identification*: the process of determining whether exposure to the hazard can cause adverse health or environmental effects.
2 *Exposure assessment*: the process of measuring and estimating the intensity, duration and frequency of human and environmental exposure.
3 *Dose–response assessment*: the process of characterizing the relationship between dose and the incidence of adverse health or environmental effects.
4 *Risk characterization*: the process of estimating the incidence of health and environmental effects under the various conditions described by the exposure assessment.

Results of the health risk assessment process are used to inform policy decisions. This policy activity is called *risk management*, and involves decisions based on judgement, in addition to the solely scientific or evidence-based results of the risk assessment process. Risk assessments can be applied to different scenarios to highlight regions or population sub-groups

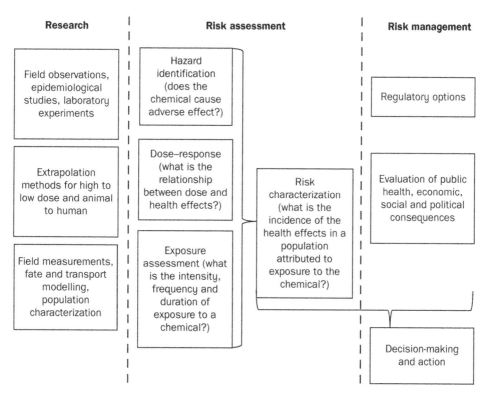

Figure 4.1 An illustration of the classical risk assessment process in relation to information inputs and contribution to decision-making.

Source: Adapted from Ball (2006).

which appear to be at higher risk. This information can then be used to inform national policy decisions for maximum health benefit.

Figure 4.1 illustrates the components of risk assessment in the field of environmental health and its relation to information inputs and contribution to decision-making.

Hazard identification

Hazard identification is an assessment of whether a substance or a product can cause harm to the environment or health. In the case of chemicals, the process examines the available scientific data for a given chemical and produces evidence to characterize the link between the exposure and its possible negative health effects. Knowledge from several scientific fields, including environmental toxicology and epidemiology, is considered and integrated in the hazard identification process.

Toxicological studies primarily involve *in vivo* testing on animals to identify hazards, including:

1 Reproductive tests to identify the effects of the chemical on reproductive performance.
2 Mutagenic tests to identify if a chemical can induce gene or chromosomal mutation in an organism.
3 Carcinogenic tests to determine if a chemical substance can cause cancer in an organism.
4 Toxicity tests to investigate the effects of a single dose (acute toxicity) or repeated doses in the short term (sub-chronic toxicity), or the effects of long-term exposure to chemicals (chronic toxicity).

Environmental epidemiological studies are used to study the distribution and causes of health states in human populations, for example to investigate the prevalence of diseases associated with chemical exposure. There are four main types of epidemiological studies:

1 Case-control studies are studies where the two comparison groups are individuals with (case) or without (control) a particular condition. These studies investigate whether there is a difference in chemical exposure between the two groups.
2 Cross-sectional studies measure the exposure to the chemical and investigate effects due to the exposure at the same point in time.
3 Cohort (longitudinal) studies follow groups of individuals and make a series of observations of both exposure and outcomes over time.
4 Ecological studies investigate exposures and outcomes in a group of people living in the same geographical area and use group measures of exposure.

Use of data from epidemiological studies is preferable to using data from toxicological studies, because there are uncertainties associated with extrapolating data from animal studies to humans. While toxicological studies can identify hazards, epidemiological studies can contribute to evidence for health effects arising from real life exposure.

The following sections discuss hazard identification and potential health effects resulting from exposure to arsenic, asbestos and POPs.

Arsenic

Arsenic is an element which is naturally occurring and widely distributed in the Earth's crust, present at an average concentration of 2 mg/kg. Acute (single, large dose) toxicity can cause death while chronic (repeated small doses) toxicity can lead to many diseases including cancers. Widespread presence of arsenic in groundwater at levels above the recommended guideline values has become a major health concern in Bangladesh, India and several other countries (see Figure 4.2)

Long-term ingestion of inorganic arsenic from water is an established cause of lung, bladder, kidney, liver and skin cancers (NRC 2001). The most clearly established non-cancer health impacts are skin changes, notably hyperkeratosis (thickening of the skin) and pigmentation changes. The evidence for other effects is strongest for hypertension and cardiovascular diseases, suggestive for diabetes and reproductive effects, and weak for cancer at sites other than lung, bladder, kidney and skin (Polya et al. 2009). Some evidence also suggests that the ingestion of arsenic may have effects on the immune and respiratory systems and pregnancy outcomes (NRC 2001).

Asbestos

Asbestos is comprised of a group of minerals that generally look like long, separable, thin fibres. Due to their fire retardant properties along with

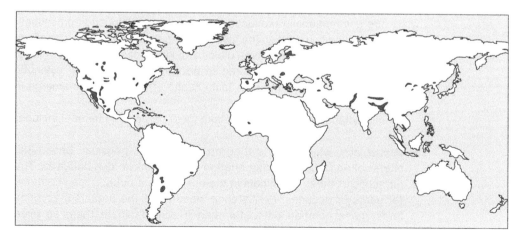

Figure 4.2 Global distribution of known major high arsenic groundwater regions in 2008.
Source: Polya et al. (2009).

resistance to chemical and biological degradation they have been extensively used in friction products, building materials and heat-resistant fabrics. Fibres of asbestos can enter into the environment from natural deposits or manufactured products. Fibres dispersed in the air can be inhaled, travel into the lungs and may cause cancer and other lung diseases.

We are all exposed to low levels of asbestos in the air (ATSDR 2001). Individuals are more likely to suffer adverse health effects when they are exposed to high levels, frequently exposed, and/or exposed for long periods, as can be the case for occupational exposures. The risk of developing lung diseases after exposure to asbestos is acutely exacerbated by smoking. The interval between exposure to asbestos and manifestation of any health effect can be as long as 40 years or more (ATSDR 2001).

The three major health effects associated with asbestos exposure are (ATSDR 2001):

- *Asbestosis*: a long-term disease of the lungs that produces progressive fibrosis of the lungs.
- *Lung cancer*: lung cancer is responsible for the largest number of deaths related to exposure to asbestos.
- *Mesothelioma*: this is a rare form of cancer that is found in the membrane of the lung, chest, abdomen and heart. Almost all cases are associated with asbestos exposure.

POPs (Persistent Organic Pollutants)

POPs are among the most hazardous compounds ever synthesized. They include pesticides (e.g. aldrin, dieldrin, endrin, dichloro-diphenyl-trichloroethane (DDT), chlordane and heptachlor) and industrial chemicals (e.g. polychlorinated biphenyls (PCBs) and polybromodiphenyl ethers (PBDEs)) that were, or are still in some countries, manufactured in great quantities. Dioxins, which are unintentionally produced by-products of combustion processes, are also included in POPs. The use of POPs has resulted in beneficial outcomes such as increased crop yields and killing pests since the 1950s. These compounds were considered to be safe chemicals until scientific information on their human and wildlife health effects began to emerge in the late 1960s and early 1970s.

The characteristics of POPs that make them particularly harmful include:

- *Persistence*, which means they are resistant to physical, photolytic, chemical and biological degradation and they have long half-lives. The presence of these chemicals in the environment or body may continue for years or decades. Persistence means that the organism accumulates these compounds faster than it can eliminate them so even small doses accumulate to measurable amounts over time (known as bioaccumulation).
- *Organic*, which means these chemicals dissolve easily in fats (lipids), i.e. they are lipophilic. Once in the environment, they are incorporated and

stored in fat tissues of animals. Thus the main source of exposure is through the food chain.
- *Pollutants*, which means they contaminate the environment and have undesired effects, such as toxic properties. Some POPs are endocrine disrupters, i.e. they are able to alter function(s) of the endocrine system (which produces hormones and has a regulatory function) and consequently cause adverse health effects (WHO 2002a, 2002b) (see also Table 4.1).
- *Persistence combined with organic* properties results in increases in body concentration of contaminants at each level in the food chain due to efficient uptake and slow elimination, i.e. they biomagnify in the food chain. Thus high concentrations of POPs can be found in large fish, fish-eating birds and mammals that eat fish.
- *Semi-volatility*, which means they evaporate into the air and therefore can travel long distances as gases.

See also Thornton (2000) for information on these harmful characteristics.

Exposure assessment

The second stage of the risk assessment process is exposure assessment. This is the process of determining the sources and routes of exposure; who is exposed, as well as measuring or estimating the intensity, frequency and duration of exposure to an agent present in the environment. There are three main routes of exposure by which chemicals in the environment can enter the body: inhalation, ingestion and dermal contact.

Table 4.1 Health effects of selected POPs

Chemical	Health effects
DDT (ATSDR 2002)	Possible carcinogen Asthma Developmental disorders including low birth weight and length Neurological disorders Endocrine disrupter
PCBs (ATSDR 2000)	Carcinogenic Chloroacne Developmental disorders Endocrine disrupter
Dioxins (ATSDR, 1998)	Carcinogenic Chloroacne Endometriosis and other fertility problems Developmental disorders Immunosupressor Liver and kidney alterations

Source: adapted from ATSDR (1998, 2000, 2002)
(see web page of ATSDR: www.atsdr.cdc.gov)

There are several different approaches for quantifying human exposure, one of which is the use of biomarkers. This is based on biochemical properties of compounds (e.g. bioaccumulation of POPs in human tissue). Levels of these biomarkers can be measured directly in blood or fat tissue samples.

Another approach is to assess the contaminant concentration in the medium to which people are exposed (e.g. water) and to use this information to estimate the intake or the dose received by individuals. Exposure assessment evaluates the rates at which the chemical crosses the boundary (chemical intake or uptake rates), the resulting amount of the chemical that actually crosses the boundary (a dose) and the amount absorbed (internal dose) (USEPA 1992). The general formula for estimating chemical intake is (adapted from Ball 2006):

$$I = (C \times IR \times EF \times ED)/BW$$

where

I = intake (µg/kg of body weight)
C = average concentration of the chemical (µg/g) during the exposed period
IR = ingestion rate (g/day)
EF = exposure frequency (days/year)
ED = exposure duration (years)
BW = body weight (kg)

Dose may be expressed as:

$$D_{pot} = C \times IR \times EF \times ED \text{ where } D_{pot} \text{ is the potential dose}$$

An average daily dose (ADD) can then be calculated by averaging D_{pot} over body weight and an averaging time, in this case per day:

$$ADD = [C \times IR \times EF \times ED]/[BW \times AT]$$

where AT is the time period over which the dose is averaged (units are days)

For effects such as cancer, where the biological response is usually described in terms of lifetime probabilities, even though exposure does not occur over the entire lifetime, doses are often presented as lifetime average daily doses (LADDs). The LADD has the same equation as ADD only with lifetime (LT) replacing the averaging time (AT):

$$LADD = [C \times IR \times EF \times ED]/[BW \times LT]$$

The following sections consider exposure assessment in relation to arsenic and POPs.

Arsenic

The most significant route of exposure to arsenic for humans who are not occupationally exposed is through the intake of food and drink (WHO 2001). Among the possible pathways of arsenic exposure illustrated in Figure 4.3, drinking water is considered the most significant. However, chronic arsenic toxicity symptoms, as recorded in Bangladesh and West Bengal (India), may reflect other exposure pathways, like soil-crop-food transfer, as well as cooking in arsenic-enriched water (Mondal and Polya 2008).

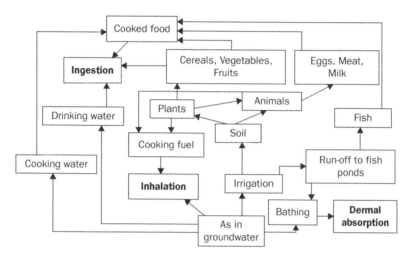

Figure 4.3 Possible routes and pathways for arsenic exposure.

Note: 'As' is the chemical symbol for arsenic.

✎ Activity 4.1

1 What is the difference between an exposure pathway and an exposure route? Find examples of each in the case of arsenic.
2 Consider arsenic exposure via groundwater for the exposed population in the Bengal delta. Compare the ADD for children and adults for a given average arsenic concentration. Assume that the typical average water consumption in this area is 2 litres per day for adults and 1 litre per day for children, and that the average adult weighs 70 kg and average child weighs 15 kg.

Feedback

1 Exposure pathway is the means by which the contaminant comes into contact with the target organism (such as arsenic contaminated drinking

water, or an arsenic contaminated crop, like rice). Exposure route is how a contaminant enters the body (such as ingestion of arsenic contaminated water or food, or dermal absorption of arsenic during bathing with arsenic contaminated water).

2 All other factors remaining equal, the ratio of child to adult ADD is as follows:

3 child: adult ADD = ((1L/day)/15kg))/((2 L/day)/70 kg)) = 2.33

In this case, the children are getting roughly twice the dose of adults despite consuming half the quantity of arsenic contaminated water. Weight for weight, children consume more food and liquids and breathe more air per kilogram of body weight than adults (Landrigan 2004).

Children are more susceptible than adults to health impacts from exposure to chemicals in the environment. Possible explanations for this include that it is due to differences in exposure (as above) or increased opportunities for exposure related to behaviour – for example, crawling on the ground and putting their hands or objects in their mouths may result in greater exposure to contaminants found in dust, carpets, soil or objects – or to differences in susceptibility:

- Children's ability to detoxify chemicals is limited because their bodies are still developing.
- Immature physiological functions make them more vulnerable to harmful health effects of chemicals.
- Children's organs are rapidly developing and growing. These developing systems are very delicate and are less able to repair damage that may be caused by toxicants than those in adults.
- As children have more years to live, they have more time to develop chronic diseases that require decades to develop and which are triggered by early exposures (Landrigan 2004).

POPs

The main source of exposure to POPs is through diet. In terrestrial ecosystems, foods such as fruits, vegetables and cereals may be contaminated with pesticides. However, due to bioaccumulation in lipids, the highest exposure is from consumption of animal fats. The animals at the top of the food chain, including humans, are the most exposed to these contaminants. The concept of bioaccumulation is illustrated in Figure 4.4, using pesticide (namely DDT) run-off into the watershed as an example.

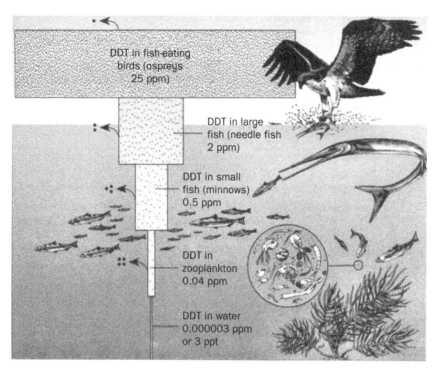

Figure 4.4 Bioaccumulation and biomagnification of DDT in the food chain.
Source: Miller (1996).

✎ Activity 4.2

1 You have read about three possible routes of exposure to environmental chemicals (ingestion, dermal contact and inhalation). What other possible routes of exposure to humans exist for these chemicals, and which particular age groups would be affected?
2 What are the policy implications for exposure to such groups?

Feedback

1 Children are additionally exposed prenatally to chemicals through the placenta and after birth through maternal milk. POPs can be transferred *in utero* from the mother to the baby. This means that a proportion of the toxins that have been accumulated in a woman's body during her life may pass through the placenta to the developing foetus in the womb and postnatally via breast milk to her children (Pronczuk et al. 2002; Barr et al. 2007). In addition, lipophilic POPs are transferred and accumulated in human milk because of its high

fat content, and such milk is the major dietary source of POPs for breastfeeding infants (WHO 2010).

2 Despite the presence of chemicals from the environment in breast milk, there is compelling evidence that breastfeeding continues to be the optimal food source for nursing infants. The benefits of breastfeeding outweigh the risks in the majority of studies (Pronczuk et al. 2002).

Most governments still recommend breastfeeding as the best option, despite potential exposures to chemicals through maternal milk. Other possible policy actions include advice to pregnant women to limit their consumption of certain food types (e.g. fish such as mackerel or salmon, which are bioaccumulators of environmental toxins), and smoked foods (to limit dioxin exposure) (NHS 2011).

Dose–response assessment

The third stage of the risk assessment process primarily aims to establish the dose or amount of the hazard that can cause damage (response) and how a change in dose will influence the likelihood or frequency of adverse health effects. If there are no epidemiological studies to provide evidence on associations between human exposures and outcomes, then the dose–response relationship is often obtained solely from toxicological studies.

Figure 4.5 shows a typical dose–response curve. Note that, for all doses above a certain dose, the maximum effect is exhibited and below this there is a range where the magnitude of the effect depends upon the dose received. For some chemicals, there is a specific dose or exposure level also known as the threshold, above which the toxic effect is produced and below which adverse effects do not occur. The threshold approach has been used to identify doses at which humans would not be expected to exhibit adverse effects. The maximum dose without effects is referred as the 'no observed adverse effect level' (NOAEL), and the lowest data point at which there is an observed toxic or adverse effect is the 'lowest observed adverse effect level' (LOAEL).

In order to obtain the tolerable daily intake (TDI), i.e. the daily dose level in which the chemical has been assessed 'safe' for humans, NOAEL and LOAEL are divided by an uncertainty factor which depends on the human or animal data available, i.e.:

TDI = NOAEL ÷ 10 (if human data) or NOAEL ÷ 100 (if animal data)
When the NOAEL is not established, the TDI= LOAEL ÷ 1000

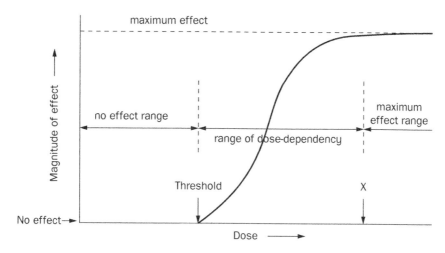

Figure 4.5 A typical dose–response curve.
Source: Ball (2006).

Note that although these are the standard factors used (WHO 2010), the figures are arbitrary and are used to afford an acceptable level of protection. These factors are based on judgement and not science. Further factors might also be incorporated depending on the severity of the health consequences of the exposure, specifically among susceptible population groups, and the quantity and quality of the scientific data on which the assessment is based (WHO 2010). For certain chemicals, notably carcinogens like arsenic, the existence of a threshold is not accepted and it is widely assumed that however small the dose is, some risk of cancer remains (Ball 2006).

There is much uncertainty in developing dose–response relationships at low doses as this relies on extrapolation of data below observed effects. For example, for arsenic, there is a clear association between arsenic exposure and various cancers at concentrations in drinking water at or above 100 µg/L, but below this concentration there is considerable uncertainty and discussion about the nature of dose–response relationships (Polya et al. 2009). The shape of the dose–response curve may vary for other chemicals and the shape is often unknown, although for non-carcinogens it is often assumed to be linear.

Risk characterization

The fourth stage in the risk assessment process is risk characterization. Risk characterization attempts to integrate the information from hazard identification, exposure assessment and dose–response assessment in order to quantify the risk to individuals, populations and/or the environment, and to provide an evaluation of the overall quality of the assessment.

The aim of risk characterization is to describe the risk to individuals or populations in terms of the nature, extent and severity of potential harm. For example, the risk of cancer from a particular contaminant is considered to be appreciable by the US Environmental Protection Agency (USEPA) if the estimated risk is greater than one person out of 10,000 having a cancer (this is a threshold to guide determination of regulatory values used by USEPA).

✎ Activity 4.3

The following figure characterizing the risk from arsenic exposure shows the cumulative probability distributions of age- and gender-adjusted excess lifetime cancer risk from rice intake, water intake and combined rice and water intake (total risk) per year for the studied population of Chakdha, West Bengal, India (Mondal and Polya 2008).

Based on the information in this figure, assess whether rice is an important pathway for arsenic exposure in the studied area, and think about the policy implications of your findings.

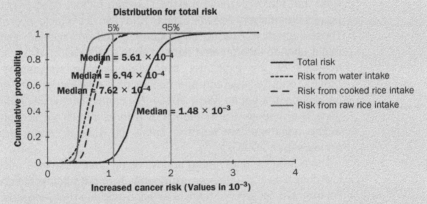

Figure 4.6 Cancer risk from rice intake, water intake and from both (total risk) per year for the population of Chakdha.

Source: Mondal and Polya (2008).

Feedback

Excess lifetime cancer risk from cooked rice intake is higher than the risk from drinking water intake for this area, suggesting that rice-related risks are of serious concern here. The estimated excess lifetime cancer risk of 7.62 per 10,000 from cooked rice intake in this area is higher than the allowable threshold for cancer risks from contaminants used by USEPA. Hence, it is important for policy-makers to plan to reduce arsenic exposure from rice intake in this area.

Risk characterization is based on a number of assumptions with varying degrees of uncertainty (USEPA 1992). Uncertainty and variability are part of every risk assessment, and need to be acknowledged and quantified in order to communicate the results clearly and unambiguously to policy-makers as well as stakeholders. Uncertainty represents a lack of knowledge about factors affecting risk characterization, whereas variability arises from true heterogeneity across people, places or time (Paustenbach 2000).

Risk characterization is also used to provide information that might be used in communicating with wider interest groups. Sometimes it is useful to compare the estimated risk from an exposure to a chemical to other health detriments of a different kind by the use of tools for comparing health states such as quality-adjusted life year (QALY) or disability-adjusted life year (DALY).

Risk management

The use of risk assessment in combination with socioeconomic and political inputs to evaluate and select measures to manage a risk is called risk management. Whereas risk assessment is based on scientific assessment, risk management is based on judgement. We will illustrate this with the example of the ratification of the Stockholm Convention on POPs.

POPs are dispersed worldwide and therefore their associated health risks cannot be managed by individual countries' regulations. Worldwide efforts have been undertaken by the UN, governments, World Health Organization (WHO) and other stakeholders in order to reduce and eliminate the production, use, trade and emission of these chemicals through the Stockholm Convention in 2001. This treaty was an international agreement by the nations of the world to protect human health and the environment against 12 POPs, known as the 'Dirty Dozen' (see Table 4.2). Most of these 12 chemicals are banned

Table 4.2 POPs listed by the Stockholm Convention

Category	The first 12 POPs	10 new POPs
Pesticides	Aldrin, chlordane, dieldrin, endrin, heptachlor, mirex, hexachrolobenzene, DDT & toxaphene	Chlordecone, α- and β-hexachlorocyclohexanes, lindane, endosulfan & pentachlorobenzene
Industrial chemicals	PCBs	Hexabromobiphenyl, perfluoroctane sulfonic, octabromodiphenyl ether & pentabromodiphenyl ether
Combustion & unintentional byproducts	Dioxins & furans	

Source: SCOPS (2011)

in high-income countries but may be in use in low- and middle-income countries (LMICs). For example, legal use of DDT is currently restricted to controlling malaria in some low-income countries.

In 2009, nine additional chemicals were added to the list of POPs, and in 2011 a further one (see Table 4.2). Many of these new chemicals are still produced and in use. Their elimination is made difficult because there may not be complete information about how to replace them, and how stakeholders may implement successful actions to reduce exposure.

In the following activity, you will be asked to apply your knowledge of risk assessment and risk management to a real-life example, to consolidate your learning for this chapter.

 Activity 4.4

Read the following description of an industrial accident that occurred in Italy in the 1970s. Think about the possible health effects (short and long term), how these would be investigated, who is at risk and what the options for control measures are.

The Seveso disaster

On 10 July 1976, an explosion at a small chemical manufacturing plant near Seveso, Italy, resulted in the highest known exposure to 2, 3, 7, 8-tetrachlorodibenzo-p-dioxin (TCDD) in the general population (Mocarelli et al. 1991). Accidental releases (technological accidents) are discussed in more detail in Chapter 10. The manufacture of TCDD was interrupted prior to finishing the final step of the process due to a law requiring shutdown of plant operations over the weekend. This led to a decomposition reaction causing the relief valve to open and up to 30 kg of TCDD was deposited over the surrounding 18 km^2 area (Di Domenico et al. 1980). TCDD is normally seen only in trace amounts (less than 1 ppm (parts per million)) (Milnes 1971). However, in the runaway reaction, TCDD production apparently reached 100 ppm or more (Hay 1979). The surrounding area was divided into four exposure zones (A, B, R, non-ABR) based on decreasing order of surface soil concentration of TCDD.

The affected community was advised not to touch or ingest vegetables or fruits from the contaminated areas. Poultry and cattle exposed to dioxins were slaughtered to prevent TCDD from entering the human food chain. A total of 3,300 animals were found dead in the following days and 15 children were hospitalized due to skin inflammation. By the end of August, Zone A had been completely evacuated and fenced. A total of 447 out of 1,600 examined people of all ages suffered from chloracne or skin lesions.

Feedback

The short-term health effects were skin lesions and in particular chloracne. The majority of cases of chloracne were diagnosed among children younger than 15 years of age. The distribution of cases was higher in Zone A, closer to the plant (Mocarelli et al. 1991).

After the incident, a health assessment of the population was initiated. As part of this effort, blood samples of some of the exposed individuals were collected and stored for chemical analyses of dioxin levels. Many studies have been performed in this area to determine the long-term health effects due to dioxin exposure. Most of these epidemiological studies have been case-control studies or longitudinal studies in which a cohort of exposed people has been followed up over time. Findings during the 20-year period following the Seveso accident showed higher risk of lymphoemopoietic neoplasm, and cancer of digestive and respiratory systems. The incidence of cancer of the thyroid gland and pleura appeared suggestively increased. In addition, dioxin exposure was associated with non-cancer effects such as endocrine effects (e.g. resulting in diabetes), cardiovascular effects and reproductive effects. Nevertheless, there are limitations in these epidemiological studies, such as small sample size for certain types of cancer and lack of individual exposure data in some (Pesatori et al. 2003). On the other hand, some of these effects have been corroborated in other studied populations exposed to dioxins and animal studies have confirmed TCDD to be a potent multi-site carcinogen as it disrupts multiple endocrine pathways (IARC 1997).

At the time of the Seveso accident, few scientific studies had reported the level of danger TCDD posed and industrial regulation was scarce. The incident gave rise to many scientific studies and standardized industrial safety regulations. The current European Union industrial safety regulation is known as the Seveso III Directive. It aimed to improve the safety of sites containing large quantities of dangerous substances as well as promote better access for citizens to information about the risks resulting from activities of nearby companies (EU 2012).

Summary

Even though many chemicals have had beneficial effects for society, their use may also produce adverse health effects. This chapter has provided an overview of the routes of environmental exposure, explored differences in vulnerability to exposure, discussed the methods used to estimate the impacts of chemicals on human health, and evaluated some of the international policies and strategies to protect human health from the exposure to chemicals. Finally, the role of environmental health risk assessment in informing risk management decisions and public health policy was discussed and illustrated with reference to POPs.

References

ATSDR (Agency for Toxic Substances and Disease Registry) (1998) *Toxicological Profile for Toxicological Profile for Chlorinated Dibenzo-p-Dioxins*. Atlanta, GA: ATSDR.

ATSDR (Agency for Toxic Substances and Disease Registry) (2000) *Toxicological Profile for PCBs*. Atlanta, GA: ATSDR.

ATSDR (Agency for Toxic Substances and Disease Registry) (2001) *Toxicological Profile for Asbestos*. Atlanta, GA: ATSDR.

ATSDR (Agency for Toxic Substances and Disease Registry) (2002) *Toxicological Profile for DDT, DDE, and DDD (2002)*. Atlanta, GA: ATSDR.

Ball, D. (2006) *Environmental Health Policy*. Maidenhead: Open University Press.

Barr, D.B., Bishop, A. and Needham, L.L. (2007) Concentrations of xenobiotic chemicals in the maternal-fetal unit, *Reproductive Toxicology*, 23(3): 260–6.

Di Domenico, A., Silano, V., Viviano, G. and Zapponi, G. (1980) Accidental release of 2, 3, 7, 8-tetrachlorodibenzop-dioxin (TCDD) at Seveso, Italy: IV. Vertical distribution of TCDD in soil, *Ecotoxicology and Environmental Safety*, 4: 327–38.

EEA (2011) http://www.eea.europa.eu/themes/chemicals, accessed 17 June 2016.

EU (2012) Seveso III Directive, Directive 2012/18/EU of the European Parliament and of the Council of 4 July 2012 on the control of major-accident hazards involving dangerous substances, amending and subsequently repealing Council Directive 96/82/EC Text with EEA relevance, http://data.europa.eu/eli/dir/2012/18/oj, accessed 16 January 2017.

European Commission (2007) *REACH in Brief* (Environment Directorate General), http://ec.europa.eu/environment/chemicals/reach/pdf/publications/2007_02_reach_in_brief.pdf, accessed 15 June 2016.

Hay, A. (1979) Seveso: the crucial question of reactor safety, *Nature*, 281(5732): 521.

Landrigan, P.J. (2004) Children as a vulnerable population, *International Journal of Occupational Medicine and Environmental Health*, 17(1): 175–7.

IARC (International Agency for Research on Cancer) (1997) Polychlorinated Dibenzo-*para*-Dioxins and Polychlorinated Dibenzofurans, *Monographs on the Evaluation of Carcinogenic Risks to Humans*, 69, http://monographs.iarc.fr/ENG/Monographs/vol69/, accessed 15 June 2016.

Miller, G.T., Jr (1996) *Living in the Environment: principles, connections and solutions*, 9th edn. Belmont, CA: Wadsworth.

Milnes, M.H. (1971) Formation of 2, 3, 7, 8-tetrachlorodibenzodioxin by thermal decomposition of sodium 2, 4, 5-trichlorophenate, *Nature*, 232(5310): 395–6.

Mocarelli, P., Marocchi, A., Brambilla, P. et al. (1991) Effects of dioxin exposure in humans at Seveso, Italy, in M. Gallo, R. Scheuplein and K. Van der Heijden (eds) *Biological Basis for Risk Assessment of Dioxins and Related Compounds*, pp. 95–110. Cold Spring Harbor, NY: Cold Spring Harbor Laboratory Press.

Mondal, D. and Polya, D.A. (2008) Rice is a major exposure route for arsenic in Chakdha Block, West Bengal: a probabilistic risk assessment, *Applied Geochemistry*, 23: 2986–97.

NHS (2011) Should pregnant and breastfeeding women avoid some types of fish?, available at http://www.nhs.uk/chq/pages/should-pregnant-and-breastfeeding-women-avoid-some-types-of-fish.aspx?nobanner=dassignup, accessed 17 June 2016.

NRC (1983) *Risk Assessment in the Federal Government: managing the process*. Washington, DC: National Academy Press.

NRC (2001) *Arsenic in Drinking Water. Update*. Washington, DC: National Academy Press.

Paustenbach, D.J. (2000) The practice of exposure assessment: a state-of-the-art review, *Journal of Toxicology and Environmental Health – Part B: Critical Reviews*, 3(3): 179–291.

Pesatori, A.C., Consonni, D., Bachetti, S. et al. (2003) Short- and long-term morbidity and mortality in the population exposed to dioxin after the 'Seveso accident, *Industrial Health*, 41(3): 127–38.

Polya, D.A., Mondal, D. and Giri, A.K. (2009) Quantification of deaths and DALYs arising from chronic exposure to arsenic in groundwaters utilized for drinking, cooking and irrigation of food crops, in V.R. Preedy and R.R. Watson (eds) *Handbook of Disease Burdens and Quality of Life Measures*. Berlin: Springer-Verlag.

Pronczuk, J., Akre, J., Moy, G. and Vallenas, C. (2002) Global perspectives in breast milk contamination: infectious and toxic hazards, *Environmental Health Perspectives*, 110(6): A349–51.

RATSC (1999) *Risk Assessment Approaches used by UK Government for Evaluating Human Health Effects of Chemicals*. The Risk Assessment and Toxicology Steering Committee, Institute for Environmental Health, UK, http://www.iehconsulting.co.uk/IEH_Consulting/IEHCPubs/IGHRC/cr2.pdf, accessed 16 January 2017.

SCOPS. Stockholm Convention on Persistent Organic Pollutants (POPs); 2011. http://chm.pops.int/Programmes/NewPOPs/The9newPOPs/tabid/672/language/en-US/Default.aspx, accessed 17 June 2016

Thornton, J. (2000) *Pandora's Poison: chlorine, health, and a new environmental strategy*. Cambridge, MA: MIT Press.

USEPA (1992) *Guidelines for Exposure Assessment*, Notice.fed.Reg 57(104), 22888-22938.

WHO (2001) Arsenic and arsenic compounds, in *Environmental Health Criteria 224*. Geneva: WHO, http://www.who.int/ipcs/publications/ehc/ehc_224/en/, accessed 10 July 2012.

WHO (2002a) Executive summary, in *Global Assessment of the State-of-the-science of Endocrine Disruptors*. International Programme on Chemical Safety. Geneva: WHO.

WHO (2002b) Introduction/background, in *Global Assessment of the State-of-the-science of Endocrine Disruptors*. International Programme on Chemical Safety. Geneva: WHO.

WHO (2010) *Persistent Organic Pollutants: impact on child health*. Geneva: WHO.

5 Water and sanitation

Rachel Peletz and Emma Hutchinson

Overview

Access to safe water and adequate sanitation are important environmental health issues, especially in low- and middle-income countries (LMICs). This chapter describes how public health interventions in relation to water, sanitation and hygiene behaviour can have substantial benefits for human health. It also discusses the implications for human health of changes in the global availability of fresh water, and evaluates policy approaches to achieve water quality which can be applied at a national level.

Learning objectives

By the end of this chapter you will be able to:

- describe the relationship between access to water, sanitation, hygiene and human health
- discuss the importance of the availability of water of sufficient quantity and quality to human health
- describe the impacts of environmental change on water and sanitation
- evaluate different criteria associated with standard-setting in relation to water quality

Key terms

Sanitation: Disposal of human excreta.

Water-based disease: Disease caused by agents that spend part of their life cycle inside an intermediate aquatic host.

Water-borne disease (faecal-oral disease): Caused by disease agents in drinking water.

Water-related vector-borne disease: Disease spread by insects that either breed in water, or are found nearby.

> **Water scarcity:** Not enough water to supply all users' needs. There are also alternative definitions that relate to per capita water availability and specific thresholds.
>
> **Water-washed disease:** Disease which could be prevented through provision of increased quantities of water.

Access to water and sanitation

Access to water is a fundamental human need, but according to the UN a third of the world's population live in countries with moderate to high 'water stress'. An area is experiencing water stress when annual water resources drop below 1,700 m^3 per person per year – the standard accepted amount per capita for meeting total water requirements, including agriculture, industry, energy and the environment (UNDP 2006). 'Water scarcity' occurs when the annual water resources drop below 1,000 m^3 per person (UNDP 2006). Then the amount of water withdrawn from lakes, rivers or groundwater is so great that resources are no longer adequate to satisfy all human or ecosystem requirements, resulting in increased competition between water users. However, domestic water use only represents a small fraction of the total requirement; it has been estimated that 50 litres per person per day (or 18.25 m^3 per person per year) is required for domestic purposes (UNDP 2006).

Access to water is not equitable. Those with the poorest access to adequate supplies of safe water tend to be communities which are already disadvantaged by poverty, such as those in peri-urban and rural areas. However, living in urban areas with adequate supplies of water available does not guarantee access; easy access to water often only reaches certain segments of the community.

Activity 5.1

A suitable quantity of water is necessary for drinking, sanitation and hygiene. Many people take access to water for granted. If you have a household supply of water, describe the situation at your home, for example:

- How many taps do you have per person?
- How many flushable lavatories are there per person?

Now consider the implications of having restricted access to water:

- Monitor your household's use of water for a day; note how many times you turn on a tap or use appliances that consume water, such as flushing the lavatory.

- What is the water being used for?
- Try to restrict yourself to one tap – preferably the one furthest away from your kitchen, outside the house if possible.
- Try to restrict your use of water.
- Consider having to do this every day and supply enough for your family.

If you don't have a household supply of water:

- consider how you get your water,
- who carries it and
- how the water is used.

Feedback

This simple activity shows how access to water can be taken for granted by those for whom it is readily available. Each household will use water in different ways and so the answers you supply will vary considerably, but by doing this you should begin to appreciate the significance access to a reliable and adequate water supply has on daily life and health.

Improved water and sanitation

One of the targets of the UN Millennium Development Goals (MDGs) was to 'halve, by 2015, the proportion of people without sustainable access to safe drinking-water and sanitation' (UN 2010). Worldwide, approximately 663 million people lacked access to improved drinking water sources and 2.4 billion people (nearly a third of the world's population) lacked access to improved sanitation in 2015 (see Figures 5.1 and 5.2). These terms are defined in Table 5.1. The type of water source was used as an approximate measure for water quality because of the logistical constraints of water quality testing and because improved drinking water sources are generally – though not always – safer than unimproved sources (Bain et al. 2014).

Time taken to access sufficient water

Though the progress of the MDGs is monitored by type of water source, 'access to water' is also dependent on the distance from a water source. Basic access is sometimes defined as having a source within 1 kilometre, or 30 minutes (walking) of a dwelling. If all of the water for a family of six people has to be carried (at least 120 litres if the requirement of 20 litres

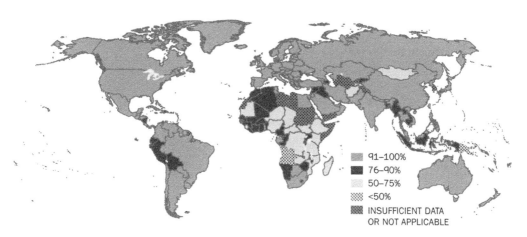

Figure 5.1 Worldwide use of improved drinking water sources in 2015.
Source: WHO/UNICEF (2015).

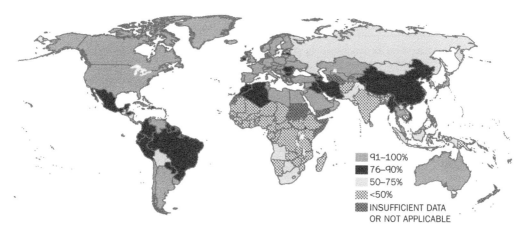

Figure 5.2 Worldwide use of improved sanitation facilities in 2015.
Source: WHO/UNICEF (2015).

per person is met), this will require many trips to ensure adequate supply. WHO estimates that a quantity of about 20 litres per capita per day should be assured to take care of basic hygiene needs and basic food hygiene (WHO 2003). Further detail on the relationship between access to water and health is presented in Table 5.2.

The journey time to collect the water, both in distance and time spent in queues, has a significant effect on water consumption (see Figure 5.3) and health (Stelmach and Clasen 2015). It is mostly women and children who are involved in water collection; freeing women from this task allows them to spend more time in other essential tasks such as improving the family income, providing opportunities for education, caring for children and preparing food.

Table 5.1 Definitions of improved water and sanitation

	Improved	Unimproved

Sanitation	Use of the following facilites:
	• Flush or pour-flush to:
	  o piped sewer system
	  o septic tank
	  o pit latrine
	• Ventilated improved pit (VIP) latrine
	• Pit latrine with slab
	• Composting toilet
		Use of the following facilities:
		• Flush or pour-flush to elsewhere (i.e. not to piped sewer system, septic tank or pit latrine)
		• Pit latrine without slab/open pit
		• Bucket
		• Hanging toilet or hanging latrine
		• Shared facilities of any type
		• No facilities, bush or field

Drinking water	Use of the following sources: • Piped water into dwelling, yard or plot • Public tap or standpipe • Tubewell or borehole • Protected dug well • Protected spring • Rainwater collection	Use of the following sources: • Unprotected dug well • Unprotected spring • Cart with small tank or drum • Tanker truck • Surface water (river, dam, lake, pond, stream, canal, irrigation channel) • Bottled water*

* Bottled water is classified as improved only when a household has access to an improved source for other purposes such as cooking and washing

Source: Modified from Joint Monitoring Programme website (http://www.wssinfo.org/definitions-methods/watsan-categories/)

Table 5.2 Summary of requirement for water service level to promote health

Service level	Access measure	Needs met	Level of health concern
No access (quantity collected often below 5 l/c/d)	More than 1000 m or 30 minutes total collection time	Consumption – cannot be assured Hygiene – not possible (unless practised at source)	Very high
Basic access (average quantity unlikely to exceed 20 l/c/d)	Between 100 and 1000 m or 5 to 30 minutes total collection time	Consumption – should be assured Hygiene – handwashing and basic food hygiene possible; laundry/bathing difficult to assure unless carried out at source	High
Intermediate access (average quantity about 50 l/c/d)	Water delivered through one tap on plot (or within 100 m or 5 minutes total collection time	Consumption – assured Hygiene – all basic personal and food hygiene assured; laundry and bathing should also be assured	Low
Optimal access (average quantity 100 l/c/d and above)	Water supplied through multiple taps continuously	Consumption – all needs met Hygiene – all needs should be met	Very low

Source: After Table S1: Summary of requirement for water service level to promote health, WHO (2003)

l/c/d = litres per capita per day

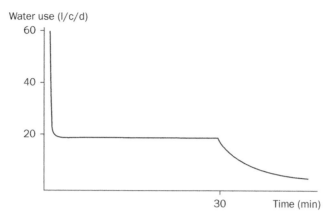

Water use (l/c/d)

Figure 5.3 Relationship between household water use and the journey time to collect water.
Source: Cairncross and Feachem (1993).

l/c/d = litres per capita per day

Table 5.3 Basic water requirements for human needs

Purpose	Litres/person/day
Drinking water	5
Sanitation	20
Bathing	15
Food preparation	10
Total	50

Source: Adapted from Gleick (1996)

It has been estimated that 50 litres per person a day are required to supply the basic requirements of an individual (Table 5.3), with an absolute minimum of 20 litres not including bathing and laundry (UNDP 2006). Insufficient water *quantity* may result in inadequate hygiene and water-washed diseases, as we will see later in this chapter.

Water quality

So far, we have mainly discussed issues related to water availability in LMICs. Another concern is the quality of the water supply. As we have seen, this can only be a relevant concern for the population if there is a sufficient quantity of water to supply people's basic needs. Water pollution (impairing quality) adds to the problem of supplying sufficient quantities because this effectively removes some of the viable water supply. Contamination may be biological, chemical, or physical, as discussed below.

An adequate water supply is essential not just for drinking and bathing, but for irrigation of crops, industry, generation of electricity, provision of sanitation and the supply of fish for food. Table 5.4 shows the wide variety of demands on the water supply, and the quality of water required for each. High water quality is only needed for drinking and cooking (potable water). The other uses for water rely on having a sufficient quantity of water; quality is less important. The protection of water sources from pollution is important to ensure a sufficient and reliable supply of acceptable water sources.

Table 5.4 Uses of water and the quality of water required

Use	Desirable quality for use	Quality after use
Water for consumption (potable water)	High quality; must meet predetermined standards	Needs treatment
Water for hygiene and sanitation	High quality not required	Needs treatment
General municipal use, fire-fighting, street-cleaning, etc.	High quality not required; many cities use the potable water supply to avoid complication	Needs treatment
Generation of electricity	Low sediment; usually uses dammed water	Reusable; there is no change to the water
Industrial	Low in sediment, mineral and biological contaminants	Mostly reusable after treatment; could be very polluted, or of high temperature if not treated
Agriculture	Not too saline or too alkaline	Polluted by pesticides, herbicides, fertilizers and salts, needs treatment for immediate reuse

Source: Adapted from Gupta and Asher (1998)

Biological contamination

Biological contamination refers to the presence of pathogens in water, also known as microorganisms or microbes. Biological contamination is the primary concern for water quality, causing the four categories of water-related diseases which will be discussed later in the chapter (water-borne, water-washed, water-based, and vector diseases). Biological contamination primarily occurs with faecal contamination and may be in the form of bacteria, viruses, helminths (worms) or protozoa.

Table 5.5 Sources of chemical constituents of water

Source	Examples
Naturally occurring	Rocks, soils and the effects of the geological setting and climate
Industrial sources and human dwellings	Mining (extractive industries) and manufacturing and processing industries, sewage, solid wastes, urban run-off, fuel leakages
Agricultural activities	Manures, fertilizers, intensive animal practices and pesticides
Water treatment or materials in contact with drinking water	Coagulants, disinfection byproducts (DBPs), piping materials
Pesticides used in water for public health	Larvicides used in the control of insect vectors of disease
Cyanobacteria	Eutrophic lakes

Source: WHO (2011a)

Chemical contamination

There is increasing public concern about the extent of water pollution due to contamination by chemicals, particularly in high-income countries. For example, the number of respondents to a Gallup poll in the USA who reported 'worrying a great deal about water pollution' was 59 per cent in 2009 (Gallup 2009). Chemical contaminants may be from natural sources or as the result of human activity. Table 5.5 describes sources of chemical contamination in water. The example of arsenic contamination is discussed in detail in Chapter 4.

Physical contamination

The physical characteristics of drinking water are usually things that can be measured with our senses: turbidity, colour, taste, smell and temperature. In general, drinking water is judged to have good physical qualities if it is clear, tastes good, has no smell and is cool. It is important to consider the physical qualities of the water that may discourage use of a particular source that is otherwise safe (in biological and chemical terms) to drink.

Water, health and disease

Having looked at the importance of quality and quantity of water, we will now move on to look in more detail at the implications for health when water is not available in sufficient quantity or quality, using a few specific examples of diseases.

Global burden of diarrhoeal disease

Faecal contamination is the world's leading avoidable environmental health problem. Over 800,000 deaths and 4 billion non-fatal cases of illness a year are attributable to diarrhoea that could be avoided through improved water supplies, sanitation and domestic hygiene (Liu et al. 2012). Inadequate drinking water and sanitation are estimated to cause 502,000 and 280,000 diarrhoea deaths per year, respectively. The most likely estimate of disease burden from inadequate hand hygiene amounts to 297,000 deaths per year. These deaths account for 1.5 per cent of the total disease burden and almost 60 per cent of diarrhoeal diseases. In children under 5 years, 361,000 deaths per year could be prevented, representing 5.5 per cent of deaths in that age group (WHO 2014a). Chemical contamination of water, despite its dramatic media coverage, does not have the same health impact. The main diseases associated with water and sanitation are summarized in Table 5.6 – they are responsible for millions of deaths and disability-adjusted life years (DALYs) every year.

Table 5.6 Global burden of water and sanitation-related disease

	Mortality estimates for 2002	DALYs 2002
Water-borne (faecal-oral)		
Diarrhoeal disease	1,798,000	61,966,000
Poliomyelitis	1000	151,000
Water-washed		
Trachoma	<1000	2,329,000
Water-based		
Schistosomiasis	15,000	1,702,000
Water-related vector		
Malaria	1,272,000	46,496,000
Lymphatic filariasis	<1000	5,777,000
Dengue	19,000	616,000
Intestinal nematode infections (helminths)	12,000	2,951,000

Source: WHO (2002)

Water-related diseases

Water affects transmission of disease in four main ways (see Cairncross and Feachem 1993):

- *water-borne:* caused by disease agents in drinking water;
- *water-washed:* disease which could be prevented through provision of increased quantities of water;

- *water-based:* caused by disease-causing agents that spend part of their life cycle inside an intermediate aquatic host;
- *water-related vector-borne:* spread by insects that either breed in water, or are found nearby.

The updated estimate of disease burden from inadequate water, sanitation and hygiene (WASH) has focused on diarrhoeal disease, and has not re-analysed the impact on other diseases which have also been associated with this risk factor, so more recent estimates than those shown in Table 5.6 are not currently available (WHO 2014a). However, the number of diarrhoea deaths attributable to inadequate water, sanitation and hygiene has dramatically reduced; falling by over 50 per cent from 1.8 million in 1990 (adjusted for comparability of methods) to 842,000 in 2012 (WHO 2014a), largely due to the efforts to meet the MDGs for water.

Water-borne disease (faecal-oral)

Water-borne transmission is the special case of ingesting faecal material in water, and any disease which can be water-borne can also be transmitted by other faecal-oral routes. There are a number of different transmission routes that allow faecal contamination to spread, as shown in the 'F-diagram' in Figure 5.4. It is difficult to identify the significance of a single transmission route, for example, drinking water, without understanding the role of the other routes such as food, flies, and unwashed fingers and others.

Preventative strategies for faecal-oral diseases include hygiene education to attempt to break cycles of transmission through these varied routes.

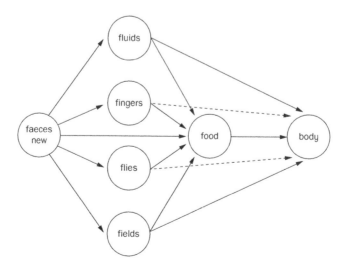

Figure 5.4 Transmission of disease from faeces: the 'F-diagram'.
Source: Wagner and Lanoix (1958).

Transmission may occur in the public domain (such as from a contaminated water supply) and in the domestic domain (such as open defecation near the household). Some examples of water-borne diseases include cholera, typhoid, shigellosis and hepatitis A and E. As water-borne diseases may also be reduced by increased provision of water, they may also be considered water-washed.

Water-washed disease

These are diseases (such as skin and eye infections and those carried by lice) that could be prevented through providing increased quantities of water for washing and cleaning.

Trachoma

The leading example of this kind of disease is trachoma, which is the consequence of eye infection with *Chlamydia trachomatis*, a microorganism which spreads through eye discharge and eye-seeking flies. There are an estimated 1.8 million people globally who are blind, visually impaired or at immediate risk of blindness from the disease and a further 55 million cases of active trachoma in need of treatment, mostly in Africa, Asia, and Central and South America (WHO 2015a). Having adequate quantities of water for washing can decrease numbers of infections by a median reduction of 25 per cent (Esrey et al. 1991).

Scabies

Scabies is a contagious skin infection that is preventable with improved personal hygiene and access to adequate water supply. Scabies is caused by the microscopic mite *Sarcoptes scabei* which burrows into the skin and deposits eggs, causing an itchy rash as an allergic response to the mites. The disease spreads through skin-to-skin contact and to a lesser extent through infested garments and bedclothes, as the presence of adequate water supply can effect a reduction in transmission by allowing washing of bedclothes. There are approximately 130 million cases of scabies worldwide each year (WHO 2014b).

Water-based diseases

Water-based diseases are those in which the disease-causing agents spend part of their life cycle inside an intermediate aquatic host; the parasites spend some of their life cycle in humans, and some inside a water-based animal. Infections are spread either through skin penetration or through ingestion. Examples of such diseases are schistosomiasis and guinea worm.

Schistosomiasis

The schistosomiasis parasite spends part of its life cycle inside snails; it then emerges into water and is able to penetrate the skin of people who are bathing or in contact with the water. There are approximately 260 million people in the world infected with schistosomiasis, of whom 20 million suffer severe consequences, including serious damage to the kidneys, liver and urinary tract. The populations most at risk are those in tropical and sub-tropical regions (WHO 2015b). Control is complex, but improved water supply helps by reducing contact opportunities with infected waters; a review of epidemiological studies found a median 77 per cent reduction in infection rates through well-designed water and sanitation interventions (Esrey et al. 1991).

Guinea worm

The guinea worm (*Dracunculus*) can only be ingested by drinking water that contains the very small crustacean *Cyclops* (the water flea), which acts as an intermediate host. The cyclops breaks down in the human stomach, releasing the worm. The female migrates through the body, emerging in a painful blister, usually in the leg, to release eggs into water, from where they return to the cyclops. The principal damage from this disease is temporary disability, both during and after the emergence of the worm.

Guinea worm is the target of an international eradication campaign. Progress has been dramatic over the past 20 years, with the number of new cases reported per year dropping from 890,000 in 1989 to 126 cases in 2014 (WHO 2015c). The disease is now found in only four countries: South Sudan, Ethiopia, Chad and Mali.

Water-related vector-borne diseases

These are diseases spread by insects that either breed in water, or are found near water. Examples of water-related vector-borne diseases include malaria, filariasis, dengue, yellow fever and onchocerciasis (river blindness). Malaria is the most significant water-related vector-borne disease, responsible for an estimated 655,000 deaths and 216 million cases per year, mostly among African children (WHO 2011b). Malaria-transmitting mosquitoes (*Anopheles*) have a wide variety of possible breeding sites, which means that water supplies make relatively little difference to malaria, except in those areas too arid to have any other year-round breeding sites. For other mosquito-transmitted diseases such as dengue, disease control may include environmental interventions to minimize standing water in order to prevent mosquito breeding, such as removal of tyre dumps which can collect water inside the tyres.

Impacts of water, sanitation and hygiene interventions on health

Types of intervention

Water quality and quantity, levels of sanitation and hygiene all contribute to the transmission of water-related diseases, and interventions exist in these areas to minimize health risks. Adequate sanitation facilities act as the primary disease barrier to prevent the spread of faecal matter. Through safe disposal of faecal matter, transmission via flies and the environment may be reduced. Good hygiene practices can further minimize transmission through contact between hands, flies, food and the environment – for example, hand washing is the single most cost-effective intervention in the spread of disease (WHO 2008). Sufficient water quantity (water supply) enables hand washing and safer food preparation, and improved water quality prevents disease transmission through contaminated drinking water. Measures may be taken to improve water quality at the source or at the household level, such as boiling or filtration.

Water and sanitation interventions include improved technologies listed previously in Table 5.1, and may be summarized by the following categories:

- water supply interventions;
- water quality interventions;
- hygiene interventions;
- sanitation interventions.

Evidence of health impact

Systematic reviews have been conducted to assess the impact of water, sanitation and hygiene interventions on health. Diarrhoea risk reductions have been assessed at 48 per cent for hand washing with soap, 17 per cent for improved water quality, 25 per cent for improved water supply and 36 per cent for excreta disposal (Esrey et al. 1985; Curtis and Cairncross 2003; Cairncross et al. 2010). Recent evidence suggests that greater reductions may be found from improvements in water quality at the household level (28–52 per cent reduction) compared to at the source (11–21 per cent reduction) (Fewtrell and Colford 2005; Waddington and Snilstveit 2009; Clasen et al. 2015) because household interventions have the potential to address recontamination during collection and storage.

It is possible that the magnitude of the actual reduction in diarrhoeal disease may be exaggerated due to reporting bias, as the majority of studies assessing household water supply were not blinded (Schmidt and Cairncross 2009), although recent studies have shown that after estimated adjustments for potential bias, interventions still reduce diarrhoeal disease by a substantial 20–48 per cent (Clasen et al. 2015).

Sanitation

Though supplying adequate quantities of safe water has the potential to reduce disease, sanitation is also essential. Inadequate sanitation increases exposure to human faeces, a risk to human health due to the pathogens they contain. Therefore the safe disposal of excreta – sanitation – is also important for maintaining environmental quality and minimizing disease risk. We consider this in more detail in this section.

Most ground- and surface water pollution in LMICs is due to inadequate sanitation. In high-income countries most sewage is collected by a municipal sewerage system, septic tank or another means. However, this does not necessarily prevent the contamination of the environment as some is pumped out to sea or into rivers or other water sources with little or no treatment. Wastewater is increasingly recycled; the reuse of grey water (wastewater from washing and cooking) has the potential to significantly cut the amounts of fresh water used for activities such as toilet flushing. 'Black water' (wastewater from toilets) is sometimes reused in agriculture because its nutrients increase production, though this will pose health risks if water is not pre-treated and workers or consumers are exposed to pathogens.

Exposure to pathogens contained in faeces is usually via contaminated drinking water, food and hands, however, helminthic worms can also enter via the skin. Pathogens associated with human faeces can cause diarrhoea, cholera, intestinal worm infections and typhoid fever. Epidemics are caused when pathogens such as *Vibrio cholorae*, which causes cholera, are introduced into areas with poor sanitation and water supply and poor food safety.

In addition to health benefits, adequate sanitation has many benefits that may be more important to the household user. One major benefit may be time-savings associated with better access, such as not having to walk long distances or wait in queues to use public facilities. In LMICs, these time savings may translate into increased production, improved education levels or more leisure time. Furthermore, sanitation has social benefits; having increased privacy may also be a motivator for households to improve sanitation. The presence of available sanitation facilities at schools may play an important role in encouraging children, and particularly girls, to continue education (due to an increase in safety). Sanitation provision may vary in urban and rural areas, and planning should take into consideration the trend of urbanization and increasing populations. Informal settlements in peri-urban areas may have developed without water and sanitation planning, and as a result may lack adequate sanitation facilities, have limited space for trucks to empty septic tanks, or result in multiple households sharing sanitation facilities, with obvious consequences for health.

Although the MDG for access to improved water has been met, the MDG targets for improved sanitation have not. Although some progress has been made, the vast majority of those without improved sanitation are poorer people living in rural areas. Progress on rural sanitation – where it has occurred – has primarily benefited the non-poor, resulting in inequalities (WHO/UN GLAAS 2014).

Environmental change and impacts on water and sanitation

A number of environmental factors, including the source of the water supply, waste disposal mechanisms and temperature, influence the spread of water-related diseases. Humidity, vegetation, crop cultivation patterns and housing quality and density are also important. Modification of habitats due to changes in patterns of water use has led to an increase in these diseases. The increasing use of irrigation and the construction of dams and reservoirs with the related changes in land use have been an important source of vector-borne disease. There is a return to support for environmental management measures to control vector-borne disease in response to the environmental and health problems associated with the use of chemical pesticides. However, including environmental management measures to protect health in water resources development projects requires action and investment from outside the health sector, including agriculture, energy, environmental agencies and local authorities, and therefore sound scientific evidence is necessary to achieve 'buy in' from these sectors so that such measures will lead to improvements in health and promote sustainability (WHO 2015d).

Climate change will affect access to clean water and adequate sanitation by increasing the risk of floods and droughts, contributing to changes in run-off that may result in water scarcity and contamination of drinking water, and therefore increase in the spread of disease. Environmental change and unsustainable consumption puts additional stress on water resources.

Water has a bearing on food security, nutrition security, poverty reduction, economic growth, energy production and human health, and as such is key to development. Increased water scarcity will result in increased competition between domestic, agricultural and industrial freshwater use as populations grow and per capita consumption increases. Without water security, there will be no food security, energy security will be compromised and poverty reduction and economic growth will not be sustainable (WHO 2015e). Because water is central to development, investing in water delivers immediate benefits as well as long-term social, economic and environmental resilience (GWP 2010a).

Environmental change and unsustainable consumption of water may also affect the Earth's water cycle. Water is an essential natural resource that shapes regional landscapes and is vital for ecosystem functioning. Human overuse of water resources, primarily for agriculture, and diffuse contamination of fresh water from urban regions and from agriculture are stressing the water resources in the terrestrial water cycle. As a consequence, the ecological functions of water bodies, soils and groundwater (e.g. filtration, natural decomposition of pollutants, buffer capacity) in the water cycle are hampered (GWP 2010b).

The Sustainable Development Goal (SDG) relating to water, SDG 6, 'ensure availability and sustainable management of water and sanitation for all', has targets to be achieved by 2030 of universal access to drinking water, adequate hygiene and sanitation, and, further to improve water quality, increase efficiency and ensure sustainable use of water. To achieve the SDGs, it is necessary to implement integrated water resources management, protect water-related ecosystems, expand infrastructure support to developing countries and strengthen participation of local communities in improving water and sanitation management (UN 2015).

Water quality guidelines and standard-setting

WHO guidelines

Water quality and treatment standards can only be defined in terms of the purpose for which water is to be used (see Table 5.3). Quality standards for treated water include setting limits for biological and chemical contamination that are a hazard to health. International guidelines for drinking water quality are produced by the WHO (WHO 2011a). For example, the WHO guidelines recommend that *E.coli* or thermotolerant coliforms should not be detectable in any 100 mL sample of water intended for drinking. These recommendations are primarily for water and health regulators, policy-makers and their advisors to assist in the development of national standards. The recommendations need to be considered in the context of managing risks from other sources of exposure, including waste, air, food and consumer products.

Approaches to standard-setting

The implementation of the WHO guidelines for drinking water quality varies among countries. There is no single approach that is used worldwide. The guidelines are recommendations to work towards and they are not mandatory limits. Countries can take the WHO guidelines into consideration along with the local environmental, social, economic and cultural conditions.

 Activity 5.2

This activity explores the implications of adopting a cost-benefit perspective on standards, as opposed to an absolutist approach of 'safe' or 'unsafe' quality. This raises the potentially controversial notion of differing standards for differing costs or populations, and the monetary or 'dollar value' of a human life. The activity will consider two strategies for water pollution management: treatment at pollutant source versus treatment before ingestion.

A water engineer has been asked to select the best options for establishing a rural water supply for a community of 200 people. She has visited the area and after some research is considering using an underground stream that emerges from a nearby hillside as the best source for the water. She is aware that groundwater is usually clean and safe. There is an alternative source available – a large river that also runs close to the village.

She takes some water samples from the underground stream and the large river and sends them to the 'Institut Pasteur' for bacteriological analysis. When the results come back, she presents them in combination with her estimates of the possible quantity of water each source can supply.

After studying the results (Table 5.7), the water engineer is initially considering two options for the supply of safe water to the village; these are set out below.

Table 5.7 Water source, bacteria count and available water

Water source	Bacteria count (E.coli/100 cm^3)	Institut Pasteur verdict	Available water (litres per person per day)
Underground stream	20	Suspected as a contamination source	20
River Styx	1000	Not fit for drinking	200

Option 1: Underground stream

Install a small treatment works which can eliminate all bacteria if properly maintained. Cost: installation US$20/person then $5/person/year cost of chemicals.

Option 2: Large river

Install sedimentation and filtration facilities before chlorination. This is required because occasionally the water is very turbid (muddy) although most of the time it is remarkably clear. Cost: installation US$200/person then $10/person/year cost of chemicals.

The engineer then receives a visit from a local environmentalist who points out that, in addition to pathogenic bacteria, there have been long-standing concerns about upstream pesticide use which may be contaminating the river water. The engineer checks the chemical content of the water for obvious contaminants, and finds 2 µg of DDT per litre of water, which lies above the recommended water quality guidelines of WHO, which are 1 µg/litre. The engineer is fortunate in that she will be able to remove the DDT from the water for the extra cost of only US$20/head/per year.

1 What issues should the engineer consider in order to choose the best option?
2 Should she take the option of removing the DDT from the river water?
3 What other policy options might the state or the pollution control authorities wish to consider?

Feedback

1 The first issue to consider is: what is the supply for the community now and what will it require in the future? You will recall that 50 litres per person per day is the minimum necessary water requirement. The problem of using the underground stream, while it has clean water, is that it may not supply a large enough quantity. One possibility may be to use it as the source of drinking water and use the river water for washing and other uses. The second issue to consider is: are there any water-related diseases causing a problem in the village already and how can they best be prevented? It may be a sanitation issue – would improved hygiene behaviour be the solution? What are the priorities for those in the village? Will the new water be of better quality than the old water? The third issue to consider is: what can the community afford to pay and where will the funds come from? How will the supply be maintained and who will pay for it?
2 It will depend partially on how much money is available and whether it is essential to use this water source or whether there are alternate sources. She might need to consider what the DDT standard is for her country.
3 The village will need to consider where the DDT is coming from and how they can control the levels. Is it possible to fine or penalize those who are allowing the DDT to enter the water supply? Are there regulations already and how can limits be enforced?

Summary

Access to water is a basic human need. The availability of both sufficient quantity and quality of water and adequate sanitation facilities varies throughout the world, but it is almost always the poorest communities who have the worst access; the technological, financial or hygiene-educational infrastructure may be inadequate, leaving them most vulnerable to water-related illness. In high-income countries water-related diseases are becoming rarer and, with increasing industrialization, chemical water pollution is the main concern. In LMICs, by contrast, water-related illnesses are the greatest source of ill health and death, although the adverse effects of unregulated industrialization are increasingly taking a toll here as well. Measures exist to regulate the quality of water. Water scarcity resulting from unsustainable consumption and climate and environmental change is a major threat to human health and future economic and social development, along with protection of the environment's provisioning services. Successful policy will require action from several sectors – agriculture, economic, energy, environmental – as well as health.

References

Bain, R., Cronk, R., Wright, J., Yang, H., Slaymaker, T. and Bartram, J. (2014) Fecal contamination of drinking-water in low- and middle-income countries: a systematic review and meta-analysis, *PLoS Med*, 11(5): e1001644, doi:10.1371/journal.pmed.1001644.

Cairncross, S. and Feachem, R. (1993) *Environmental Health Engineering in the Tropics*, 2nd edn. Chichester: John Wiley & Sons Ltd.

Cairncross, S., Hunt, C., Boisson, S. et al. (2010) Water, sanitation and hygiene for the prevention of diarrhoea, *International Journal of Epidemiology*, 39: i193–i205.

Clasen, T.F., Alexander, K.T., Sinclair, D. et al. (2015) Interventions to improve water quality for preventing diarrhoea, *Cochrane Database of Systematic Reviews*, 10, Art. No.: CD004794, doi: 10.1002/14651858.CD004794.pub3.

Curtis, V. and Cairncross, S. (2003) Effect of washing hands with soap on diarrhoea risk in the community: a systematic review, *Lancet Infectious Diseases*, 3: 275–81.

Esrey, S.A., Feachem, R.G. and Hughes, J.M. (1985) Interventions for the control of diarrhoeal diseases among young children: improving water supplies and excreta disposal facilities, *Bulletin of the World Health Organization*, 63(4): 757–72.

Esrey, S.A., Potash, J.B., Roberts, L. and Shiff, C. (1991) Effects of improved water supply and sanitation on ascariasis, diarrhoea, dracunculiasis, hookworm infection, schistosomiasis, and trachoma, *Bulletin of the World Health Organization*, 69(5): 609–21.

Fewtrell, L. and Colford, J.M., Jr (2005) Water, sanitation and hygiene in developing countries: interventions and diarrhoea – a review, *Water Science & Technology*, 52(8): 133–42.

Gallup (2009) Gallup Environmental Survey, www.Gallup.com/poll/117079/water-pollution-Americans-Top_Green-Concern.aspx, accessed 7 November 2015.

Gleick, P.H. (1996) Basic water requirements for human activities: meeting basic needs, *Water International*, 21(2): 83–92.

Gupta, A. and Asher, M. (1998) *Environment and the Developing World: principles, policies and management*. Chichester: John Wiley & Sons Ltd.

GWP (Global Water Partnership) (2010a) The urgency of water security, http://www.gwp.org/en/The-Challenge/The-Urgency-of-Water-Security, accessed 11 November 2015.

GWP (Global Water Partnership) (2010b) Water resources management, http://www.gwp.org/en/The-Challenge/Water-resources-management/, accessed 11 November 2015.

Liu, L. et al. (2012) Global, regional, and national causes of child mortality: an updated systematic analysis for 2010 with time trends since 2000, *Lancet*, 379(9832): 2151–61.

Schmidt, W.P. and Cairncross, S. (2009) Household water treatment in poor populations: is there enough evidence for scaling up now?, *Environmental Science & Technology*, 43(4): 986–92.

Stelmach, R.D. and Clasen, T.F. (2015). Household water quantity and health: a systematic review, *International Journal of Environmental Research and Public Health*, 12(6): 5954–5974, doi:10.3390/ijerph120605954.

UN (2010) Fact sheet No. 35, *The Right to Water*. New York: UN.

UN (2015) Sustainable Development Goals, https://sustainabledevelopment.un.org/?menu=1300, accessed 11 November 2015.

UNDP (United Nations Development Program) (2006) *Human Development Report 2006: beyond scarcity: power, poverty and the global water crisis*. New York: UNDP, http://hdr.undp.org/en/media/HDR06-complete.pdf.

Waddington, H. and Snilstveit, B. (2009) Effectiveness and sustainability of water, sanitation, and hygiene interventions in combating diarrhoea, *Journal of Development Effectiveness*, 1(3): 295–335.

Wagner, E.G. and Lanoix, J.N. (1958) *Excreta Disposal for Rural Areas and Small Communities*. Geneva: WHO.

WHO (2002) *World Health Report: Reducing Risks, Promoting Healthy Life*. Geneva: WHO.

WHO (2003) *Domestic Water Quantity, Service Level and Health*, http://www.who.int/water_sanitation_health/diseases/WSH0302exsum.pdf?ua=1), accessed 11 November 2015.

WHO (2008) *Global Handwashing Day 15 October: Planner's Guide*, http://www.who.int/gpsc/events/2008/Global_Handwashing_Day_Planners_Guide.pdf, accessed 15 November 2015.

WHO (2011a) *Guidelines for Drinking-water Quality*, 4th edn. Geneva: WHO.

WHO (2011b) *World Malaria Report*, http://www.who.int/malaria/world_malaria_report_2011/en/.

WHO (2014a) Preventing diarrhoea through better water, sanitation and hygiene: exposures and impacts in low- and middle-income countries, http://apps.who.int/iris/bitstream/10665/150112/1/9789241564823_eng.pdf?ua=1, accessed 11 November 2015.

WHO (2014b) Scabies, http://www.who.int/lymphatic_filariasis/epidemiology/scabies/en/, accessed 17 November 2015.

WHO/UN GLAAS (2014) Investing in water and sanitation: increasing access, reducing inequalities (UN-Water Global Analysis and Assessment of Sanitation and Drinking-Water). Geneva: WHO, http://apps.who.int/iris/bitstream/10665/143953/2/WHO_FWC_WSH_14.01_eng.pdf.

WHO (2015a) Trachoma factsheet, no. 382, http://www.who.int/mediacentre/factsheets/fs382/en/, accessed 17 November 2015.

WHO (2015b) Schistosomiasis factsheet, no. 115, http://www.who.int/mediacentre/factsheets/fs115/en/, accessed 17 November 2015.

WHO (2015c) Dracunculiasis (guinea-worm disease) factsheet, no. 359, http://www.who.int/mediacentre/factsheets/fs359/en/, accessed 17 November 2015.

WHO (2015d) *Water, Sanitation, Health: Environmental Management for Vector Control*, http://www.who.int/water_sanitation_health/resources/envmanagement/en/, accessed 11 November 2015.

WHO (2015e) *Water Supply, Sanitation and Hygiene Development*, http://www.who.int/water_sanitation_health/hygiene/en/, accessed 11 November 2015.

WHO/UNICEF (2015) *Progress on Drinking Water and Sanitation 2015 Update*. Geneva: WHO/UNICEF Joint Monitoring Programme for Water Supply and Sanitation.

6 | Housing and indoor environment

James Milner and Emma Hutchinson

Overview

The quality of the environment inside our homes is important for maintaining good health. It is affected by how we cook and prepare food; how our homes are built and maintained; how service utilities are provided; how homes are heated and whether they are overcrowded. This chapter gives an overview of all these aspects with particular focus on air pollution, overcrowding, heat and cold and the rising importance of indoor air pollution (or household air pollution) in low- and middle-income countries (LMICs). Other risk factors such as accidents and falls in the home are outside the scope of this chapter.

Learning objectives

By the end of this chapter you will be able to:

- describe health issues associated with poor housing
- discuss hazards associated with the quality of the indoor environment and their relative impact on human health in low- and high-income countries
- evaluate the methods used to estimate the burden of disease from household air pollution
- discuss current policies to ensure 'healthy housing'

Key terms

Biomass fuel: Organic material, such as animal dung, wood or crop residues which may be burned as a fuel.

Energy efficiency: The percentage of the total energy input that is consumed in useful work rather than lost as heat. For heating systems, efficiency may also refer to the proportion of generated heat that is captured for heating the home.

Excess cold (or heat): Temperatures too low (or high) to maintain health, comfort and wellbeing. Excess cold or heat depends not only on temperature but also on other factors such as the level of activity of the individual and their clothing.

Fuel poverty: A situation in which householders would have to spend a high proportion of their income on heating and other fuel costs to keep adequately warm at reasonable cost, given their income. In the UK, fuel poverty is now defined as occurring when a household's required fuel costs are above the national median level, and at that level of expenditure the household would be left with a residual income below the official poverty line (Hills 2012).

Ventilation: The replacement of indoor air with 'fresh' air – either from outdoors or from circulation of air within the building.

The relationship between the indoor environment and health

This chapter is concerned with the quality of the indoor environment, particularly in the home, and its impact on health. Occupational settings, such as schools and the workplace, are also very important but these are not the primary focus of this chapter. The indoor environment should also be seen in relation to the outdoor environment because indoor air pollution is dependent, to some extent, on the level of outdoor pollution; waste is removed from the home and housing is situated within a physical and social community, which may have a bearing on the indoor environment. For example, homes located on busy roads will have higher concentrations of air pollutants derived from traffic sources, and perceptions of risk and danger such as fear of crime and feelings of safety and security may be affected by the level of social cohesion in any particular area. These issues are discussed further in Chapter 9 on the urban environment and health.

Improving the indoor environment, especially in housing, has long been a key area for improving health. As early as the nineteenth century, authorities in countries such as the UK began to target sanitation and overcrowding to reduce the spread of infectious diseases. Opportunities to improve health through better housing are important because people spend a high proportion of their time in the home. In high-income settings, people spend on average over two-thirds of their time in the home, and this proportion rises for many vulnerable sub-groups, such as children and the elderly (EPA 2011).

Activity 6.1

There are many different ways in which the indoor environment may adversely affect human health. The indoor domestic environment varies widely both within and between countries. Homes in countries at different stages of development will experience very different indoor environmental hazards. These hazards may also vary by the wealth of householders, geographical location, construction methods, level of provision of services and many other factors.

Make a list of hazards associated with the indoor environment and how these might influence health in (1) high- and (2) low- and middle-income countries.

Feedback

Table 6.1 gives examples of a few of the hazards you might have thought of.

Table 6.1 Selected hazards of the indoor environment and example impacts on health

Hazard	Example health outcomes
Cold (mainly temperate climates)	Cardio-respiratory illness
Falls, accidents	Physical injury
Damp, mould	Respiratory illness
Poor indoor air quality	Respiratory illness, lung cancer
Poor sanitation	Diarrhoea, vector-borne disease
Overcrowding	Spread of infectious disease

Although different hazards may be more or less prevalent in high-, middle- or low-income countries, there is no clear division. Most hazards are relevant in all three settings. For example, overcrowding is a common problem in LMICs, but it may also be a problem among some groups in high-income countries; and damp and mould are also problems in LMICs as well as in high-income countries. Lack of adequate water supplies and sanitation in LMICs leads to substantial health burdens from diarrhoea, and from vector-borne disease, such as malaria, which is a major risk in tropical and sub-tropical climatic zones (see Chapter 5).

Aspects of housing and health

Housing can affect health, both positively and negatively, in a number of ways. For example, health may be influenced by the building's design and construction, the energy sources used for heating and cooking, and how the building is used by the people within it. These factors may also interact with the social conditions of the occupants.

Building design- and construction-related problems

Many countries have set enforceable standards for the design and construction of buildings to help protect health and safety. These cover such things as ventilation characteristics, levels of thermal insulation, fire and accident risks. However, in many settings the monitoring and enforcement of building standards are ineffective or they do not exist. Particular problems may arise with informal settlements or slum developments, which often carry particularly high risks of fire, explosion, collapse, accidents and pollution. Dwellings in informal settlements are also often vulnerable to the effects of natural disasters, such as high winds, landslides and earthquakes.

Building materials themselves may be harmful – asbestos was widely used (chiefly as a fire retardant) in commercial and domestic buildings as well as schools and hospitals. It has now been shown to be a harmful material that causes lung cancer, mesothelioma and other illnesses (Mølhave et al. 2004).

Accidents in the home are a leading cause of injury worldwide. Overcrowding, poor design and maintenance, and use of poor quality materials contribute to accident risks. For example, poorly designed buildings and fittings can lead to falls, particularly in the elderly and young children. If shelters are made of flammable materials, or cooking fires and stoves are unsafe, the risk of death and injury due to fire is increased. Poor design in the layout of the room can lead to inadequate space and ventilation for cooking, and problems with hygiene.

The indoor environment also has an impact on mental health. For example, poor quality housing, overcrowding and the threat of flooding can all influence the mental health of inhabitants.

Housing, hazards and indoor air quality

Table 6.2 summarizes some of the major hazards typically found in a home in a high-income country setting and was used to establish the UK's Housing Health and Safety Rating System (HHSRS) (Office of the Deputy Prime Minister 2006), a tool used to grade the danger from selected housing hazards. The health risks associated with a given dwelling type are assessed on the basis of the individual hazards and their collective probability of causing harm.

Indoor air quality is a specific hazard of the indoor environment with a wide range of determinants. Levels of pollutants are strongly affected by the behaviour of building occupants, for example their use of cleaning materials, window opening (and thus levels of ventilation), cooking methods (particularly the use of biomass in low- and middle-income settings), use of heating appliances (type and quality of maintenance) and smoking. Some of the main pollutants in indoor environments include:

- *Particulate matter (especially fine particulate matter)*: which has been linked to all-cause, cardiopulmonary and lung cancer mortality in epidemiological studies (e.g. Pope et al. 2002). Although much of the current

Table 6.2 Range of housing-related hazards

Category	Type	Hazards
Physiological requirements	Hygrothermal conditions	Damp and mould growth; excess cold; excess heat
	Pollutants (non-microbial)	Asbestos (and manufactured mineral fibres (MMF)); biocides; carbon monoxide and fuel combustion products; lead; radiation; uncombusted fuel gas; volatile organic compounds
Psychological requirements	Space, security, light and noise	Crowding and space; entry by intruders; lighting; noise
Protection against infection	Hygiene, sanitation and water supply	Domestic hygiene, pests and refuse; food safety; personal hygiene, sanitation and drainage; water supply
Protection against accidents	Falls	Falls associated with bathrooms etc.; falling on the level surfaces etc.; falling on stairs etc.; falling between levels
	Electric shocks, fires, burns and scalds	Electrical hazards; fire; flames, hot surfaces etc.
	Collisions, cuts and strains	Collision and entrapment; explosions; position and operation of amenities etc.; structural collapse and falling elements

Source: Office of the Deputy Prime Minister (2006)

evidence of the adverse health effects of air pollution is based on studies in relation to outdoor air pollution, there is a growing body of literature about pollution from indoor sources, especially the use of biomass burning without adequate ventilation.

- *Nitrogen dioxide (NO$_2$)*: which has been especially associated with respiratory disease.
- *Carbon monoxide (CO)*: a clear, odourless gas which can be released into homes by faulty or poorly maintained boilers and other gas appliances, such as cookers, grills, etc. Failure of such appliances, combined with poor ventilation, can lead to levels that are fatal.
- *Radon:* a radioactive gas which seeps into homes through the floor, especially in areas with predisposing geology and soil (containing high levels of elements in the uranium or thorium series). Radon is the second most important risk factor for lung cancer after smoking (National Cancer Institute 2011).
- *Environmental tobacco smoke (ETS):* sometimes referred to as second-hand smoking or passive smoking, ETS exposure in non-smokers has been linked to increased risk of lung cancer, heart attack, heart disease and stroke (e.g. Law et al. 1997; Lee and Forey 2006).

Table 6.3 Common indoor air pollutants and sources

Pollutant	Sources
Nitrogen dioxide (NO_2)	Heating and cooking appliances
Carbon monoxide (CO)	Heating and cooking appliances
Particulate matter (PM)	Cooking and aerosols
Radon	Ground gases especially in defined areas
Environmental tobacco smoke (ETS)	Cigarettes, cigars and pipes
Allergens	Moulds and house dust mites
Volatile organic compounds and ozone	Cleaning products, paints and printers

Source: Adapted from UK Parliament (2010)

The sources of these and other household air pollutants (HAPs) are summarized in Table 6.3. It is important to appreciate sources of HAPs in order that measures can be taken to reduce or control them.

The indoor environment can be polluted from sources originating outdoors as well as from those inside the home, as we have seen. Pollution from outside sources includes a variety of mainly traffic-related and industrial sources (see Chapter 7). Ventilation helps to remove pollutants generated indoors but also allows pollution from the outdoor air to enter into indoor environments. In high-income settings, there has been a move in recent years to try to reduce energy consumption in houses by minimizing ventilation rates in order to limit uncontrolled heat losses. As you will see later, ventilation also plays a key role in regulating indoor temperatures and controlling moisture and damp (by its effect on improving air exchange). However, several studies have found that reducing ventilation too much can lead to negative health effects arising from increased concentrations of air pollutants and favourable conditions for mould growth (e.g. Jacobs et al. 2009). There is therefore a potentially important trade-off between energy efficiency and health.

Overcrowding

Overcrowding is a common hazard in all countries which causes and exacerbates a number of health problems. Although there is no universally accepted definition, overcrowding often occurs as a result of traditional multigenerational family units living together in houses designed for smaller families. It is commonly associated with poverty and is the result of necessity rather than choice. When conditions become crowded there is increased risk of transmission of infectious diseases such as influenza, meningitis, diarrhoea and tuberculosis, and of accidents. As a result of poverty, diet in these households is often poor, and malnutrition can increase the susceptibility of inhabitants. Overcrowding is also associated with violence and stress-related mental health disorders. The effects of psychological stress are important, particularly for women who may be at greater risk of this type of stress, as they often spend more time in the home environment than men. Children are also particularly vulnerable to the diseases and stresses of overcrowding because of the time they spend in the home, and having little room to play or study can negatively impact on their development (Krieger and Higgins 2002; Office of the Deputy Prime Minister 2004).

Indoor temperature and health

Temperature within dwellings is an important factor for health. Excess cold or heat is associated with an increase in mortality and morbidity. The effects of temperature on health are likely to be modified by housing conditions such as the level of thermal insulation and the efficiency of heating and cooling systems. During the August 2003 heatwave, 15,000 excess deaths were observed in Paris, with over twice that number across western Europe as a whole. Factors associated with heat-related mortality and morbidity during this heatwave were reported to include poor thermal properties of dwellings and sleeping on the top floor of the building. Elderly people were particularly affected due to lack of mobility and pre-existing medical conditions (Vandentorren et al. 2006). It is likely that the public health impact may have been less if an emergency plan for high temperatures had been in place, enabling preventative action to have been taken more quickly. The role of emergency planning in the health care system is discussed in Chapter 10, and the improvements that have since been made to emergency planning specifically for heatwaves in Chapter 12.

In temperate climates, health is also adversely affected by living in cold homes. Interventions targeting thermal comfort have been shown to improve both physical and mental health (Green and Gilbertson 2008).

 Activity 6.2

Read the following short extract on cold houses and excess winter mortality in elderly people from Wilkinson et al. (2004). Having read the extract and accompanying text, explain how you would target interventions to prevent cold-related winter excess mortality in elderly people and maximize the improvement in public health.

Cold houses and excess winter mortality in elderly people

In the United Kingdom mortality greatly increases in winter. This is apparent at all ages but is greatest in relative and absolute terms in elderly people. Much of the excess seems to be related to cold, yet Britain has a larger seasonal fluctuation in mortality than many other countries of continental Europe and Scandinavia despite having milder winters. Behavioural factors may partly explain this, but poor housing may also be important.

To investigate this, the authors studied mortality in people aged over 75 years, focusing on individual determinants of vulnerability, including socioeconomic factors, sex, home heating and previous health. The study found that:

*   most of the seasonal fluctuation in mortality was related to cold, with smaller components attributable to influenza A and other risk factors (Figure 6.1);
*   the overall winter:non-winter rate ratio for daily mortality was 1.31;
*   there was no evidence that socioeconomic deprivation or self-reported financial worries were predictive of winter death;
*   female sex and a history of respiratory illness may confer vulnerability;
*   the risk of winter death was widely distributed in elderly people rather than being heavily concentrated in the most disadvantaged groups.

There was little evidence that this ratio varied by geographical region, age or any of the personal, socioeconomic or clinical factors examined, with two exceptions: after adjustment for all major covariates the winter:non-winter ratio in women compared with men was 1.11 (1.00 to 1.23), and those with a self-reported history of respiratory illness had a winter:non-winter ratio of 1.20 – 1.08 to 1.34 times that of people without a history of respiratory illness.

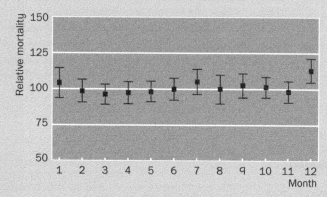

Figure 6.1 Fraction of deaths attributable to monthly variation (adjusted for region, time trend, month, low temperature and influenza). Relative mortality (y-axis) defined as mortality in winter (December to March) relative to mortality in non-winter periods.
Source: Wilkinson et al. (2004).

Apart from these exceptions, there was little evidence for vulnerability to winter death being associated with factors thought to lead to vulnerability. The authors concluded that public health policies to reduce the burden of winter death in Britain will need to be broad-based and to consider measures additional to those aimed at tackling fuel poverty.

Feedback

The study found that most of the seasonal fluctuation in mortality was related to cold with a 31 per cent increase in winter mortality relative to the rest of the year. This study in particular provided no clear evidence of effect modification by housing type. While some reasonably argue that housing is a major factor in vulnerability to cold, it is not a conclusion that can be drawn from this paper. There are those who continue to argue that it is exposure in the outdoor environment which is critical.

To decrease the number of winter deaths, any intervention has to be targeted at the population most likely to benefit. Wilkinson et al. (2004) suggest the most vulnerable groups may be elderly women and those with a history of respiratory illness, but that the risks are widely distributed in the population.

It is not just living in energy-inefficient housing that is the cause of low internal temperatures; fuel poverty is another important factor. It can mean people are unable to heat their homes adequately without compromising expenditure in other areas. Tackling fuel poverty would suggest targeting those on low incomes. However, the results of this study showed a lack of socioeconomic gradient in excess winter mortality. This has implications for public health policies aimed at reducing the burden of winter death, as fuel poverty relief alone may be only partially successful. The fact that the risk of excess winter death seems to be widely distributed in elderly people suggests that additional measures are needed to reach all those at risk.

Damp housing

Cold homes are more likely to lead to the presence of damp. Levels of damp within homes are also influenced by other factors including the rate of internal moisture generation (dependent on occupancy), ventilation, surface materials and ingress of water from outside. Some studies have suggested that up to 50 per cent of buildings in Europe and North America may be affected to some extent (Mudarri and Fisk 2007). Damp, cold conditions provide an ideal environment for mould growth, which has been consistently linked to a number of respiratory illnesses such as asthma, wheeze, cough, respiratory infection and upper respiratory tract symptoms. A meta-analysis of 33 studies by Fisk et al. (2007) estimated that building dampness and visible mould growth are associated with a 30–50 per cent increase in the risk of a variety of respiratory- and asthma-related health outcomes, with severity increasing with increasing levels of damp and mould in the home. The effects have been observed in studies conducted in many geographical regions and for different age groups, though there is particular concern over the impacts in infants and children. There is also a link with socioeconomic deprivation; housing that is damp and prone to condensation tends to be poorly maintained.

Household air pollution in LMICs

Household air pollution (HAP) in LMICs has been identified as one of the most important environmental global concerns today. About half of the world's population (3 billion) use biomass or solid fuels to provide energy for cooking and heating. If burned without being vented to the outside (and often using inefficient stoves), these fuels can be a major source of indoor particulate concentrations. Globally, 4.3 million deaths were attributable to household air pollution exposure in 2012, almost all in LMICs (see Figure 6.2 for regional-specific death rates).

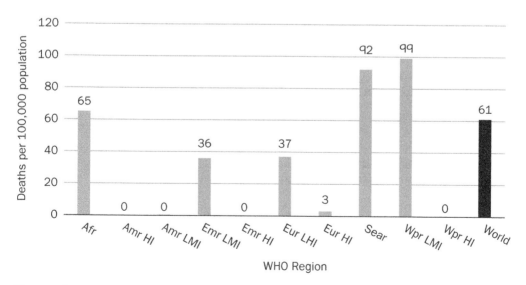

Figure 6.2 Deaths attributable to household air pollution (HAP) in 2012, by WHO region.
Notes: Amr: America; Afr: Africa; Emr: Eastern Mediterranean; Sear: South-East Asia; Wpr: Western Pacific; LMI: low and middle income; HI: high income.
Source: Figure 2 (WHO 2014a).

Recent estimates of the global burden of disease (GBD) from household air pollution from solid fuels also suggest that this specific exposure accounts for a significant proportion of global morbidity, with the absolute number of disability-adjusted life years (DALYs) accounted for by solid fuel exposures in 2010 worldwide estimated at 94.6 million, with 33.7 million of these in men, 21.8 million in women and 39.1 million in children (Smith et al. 2014). Respiratory infections account for around 40 per cent of the total global burden of disease from household air pollution for mortality, while cardiovascular disease accounts for 60 per cent (WHO 2014a).

Women and children are the groups most likely to be in close proximity to this source of pollution, due to the time that they spend indoors. Personal exposure estimates derived by the WHO indicate that women experience higher personal exposure levels than men and therefore potentially a higher relative risk to develop adverse health outcomes due to their greater involvement in daily cooking activities. However, the absolute burden is larger in men due to larger underlying disease rates in men (WHO 2014a).

Open fires for cooking and heating are common in both rural and peri-urban areas. The fire is usually at floor level, often with a tripod or bricks on which to rest cooking pots; in addition to the pollution it produces, this design can result in accidents and problems with food hygiene. There is often no chimney to remove smoke and, as biomass fuels often burn inefficiently, there are high levels of particulates and other pollutants in comparison with other fuel sources. Burning of solid fossil fuels such as coal can lead to similar problems, particularly if the fuel is of poor quality and burns inefficiently. The indoor concentration of health-damaging pollutants from a typical wood-fired cooking stove creates carbon monoxide and other noxious fumes at anywhere between 7 and 500 times the allowable limits, far exceeding international safety standards.

Indoor air pollution in India

India relies heavily on the use of biomass fuels for cooking and heating. The WHO estimates that 82 per cent of people in India cook using solid fuel and almost half a million deaths each year are the result of the indoor pollution produced by these sources of particulates, mainly from acute lower respiratory infection in children (WHO 2009).

Activity 6.3

Read the extract below by Smith (2000) on the burden of disease attributable to household air pollution in India. What difficulties did the author highlight in using epidemiological studies to understand the burden of household air pollution in LMICs?

National burden of disease in India from household air pollution

If verified, the ill health estimated here from indoor air pollution is a substantial portion of the national total in India, 4.2–6.1%. It is equivalent to 6.3–9.2% of the burden for women and children under 5, who make up about 44% of the population but bear about two-thirds of the disease burden . . . indoor air pollution would seem to classify as a major cause of ill health in India for it rivals or exceeds Tuberculosis, Ischemic Heart Disease, all cancers, road accidents, or all of the 'tropical' diseases combined. On a risk factor basis, the burden of dirty air at the household level lies behind only dirty water at the household level (poor water/sanitation/hygiene = 10%) and poor food at the household level (malnutrition = 22%), the largest two risk factors in India in the early 1990s . . . it apparently substantially exceeded other major risk factors, such as hypertension, alcohol, unsafe sex, and tobacco . . . by any standard, indoor air quality would seem to be a major health issue in the country. Adding urban outdoor pollution, the total would be even greater. Taking the dubious but simple approach of adding the estimates, the total annual deaths would be 600,000–750,000. Assuming a similar mix of morbidity and mortality, the total burden from air pollution in India would be 5.9–9.2% of the total NBD (National Burden of Disease), nearly rivalling poor water/sanitation/hygiene, although still well below malnutrition.

Discussion and conclusion

At the global level, India seems to have some 30% of all household solid-fuel stoves, although the estimates are generally much less reliable than in India where fuel use is determined in the national census. On that basis, the total world health impact on women and children would be roughly three times larger than the Indian estimates. A large fraction undoubtedly occurs in China, where application of broad-brush methods have also derived large health impacts of indoor and outdoor pollution with relatively more Chronic obstructive airways disease and lung cancer and less Acute Respiratory Infection than found in India. . . By themselves, epidemiological studies do not prove causality, only association. Nevertheless, when a number of studies find similar associations in different populations, places, and times; in situations of different mixes of confounders; and done by different investigators with different methods; the argument for causality starts to become stronger. The studies in less developed country solid-fuel-using households reviewed here have generally not directly measured exposures, nor have they been as nearly as extensive or sophisticated as those in developed-country urban settings. Nevertheless, particularly for the diseases above, a number of studies have been done by different investigators in different countries that found similar results. Combined with the evidence that the average particle levels in such households often reach 1 000–2 000 μg/m^3 PM$_{10}$, their results seem qualitatively consistent with the developed-country studies, which have been done at levels below 150 µg/m. On the other hand, given that most actually measured the risk of solid fuel use, there may be risks to health in addition to air pollution, perhaps through the physical burden of harvesting such fuels. The estimates made here should be viewed as tentative. They rely on distressingly few studies and many untested assumptions. Their alarming scale, however, argues for additional efforts to understand and ameliorate the conditions that lead to such severe pollution levels in the village and urban slum homes of India and elsewhere in the developing world.

Feedback

The national burden of disease in India from indoor pollution has been indirectly estimated by calculation, combining data on exposures, exposure-response functions and background disease rates. The author points out that epidemiological studies can point to association, but not causality. However, the mounting evidence from different regions and countries strengthens the argument for the existence of a link between household air pollution and ill health. Other potential difficulties in assessing the disease burden were:

- exposure was not directly measured, unlike studies on outdoor pollution in high-income countries (see Chapter 7);
- where indoor exposures have been measured, they are much greater than those in outdoor studies in high-income countries;
- any estimate of the burden of disease from biomass fuel should also take into consideration the added risks from the physical burden of harvesting or collecting the biomass fuel;
- the estimates in this study come from only a few cases with untested assumptions;
- the problem is large in scale and more research should be done to ascertain the impact on health.

Since the Smith (2000) study, further research has been conducted on the impacts of household air pollution on health, with suggestive evidence for pneumonia (Smith et al. 2011) and other health effects including respiratory illness, lung cancer, chronic obstructive pulmonary disease (COPD), weakening of the immune system and decreased lung function (Zhang and Smith 2007). Further work has also been conducted on exposure assessments, highlighting kerosene as an important contributor to household air pollution (Bates et al. 2013). Although solid fuel use is declining in some regions, due to population growth the absolute impact is not declining, with some regions (in particular Africa) experiencing a substantial increase in solid fuel use over the last 30 years (77 per cent of households in 2010, representing 646 million people exposed) (Bonjour et al. 2013).

Strategies for improving health in the indoor environment

We have seen in this chapter that at the global level the highest priorities for improving health in the indoor environment include addressing indoor air pollution from unvented and inefficient biomass burning, as well as improving water supply and sanitation (as discussed in Chapter 5). In higher income countries, the priorities are on energy efficiency and in reducing consumption of energy (discussed later in the chapter). In all regions, quality and appropriateness of construction to the local environment (e.g. suitable building construction in earthquake prone areas) is also important.

Reducing household air pollution from biomass fuels

In 2009, through the National Biomass Cookstove Initiative, India set a goal of achieving 'a quality of energy services from cookstoves comparable to that from other clean energy sources such as LPG' (liquefied petro-leum gas) (Ministry of New and Renewable Energy 2009). A number of other countries have launched similar programmes, which will require a combination of policy and technological interventions. The UN has also established the Global Alliance for Clean Cookstoves which uses public and private funding towards achieving the goal of universal adoption of clean cookstoves and fuels (UN Foundations 2012). However, there is some evidence that substituting traditional technology with modern inno-vations can result in continued or even increased pollution from new sources (Kar et al. 2012).

Some technological methods for reducing exposure to indoor particulates are listed below.

- *Change fuel type*: processed fuels and biogas are less polluting than raw fuel but are more expensive.
- *Change stove type*: use technology to improve energy efficiency of the stove or heater – there are relatively inexpensive alternatives available (Figure 6.3 gives an example).
- *Separate cooking from other activities*: however, if space is limited, this might not be possible.
- *Reduce exposure by improving ventilation*.
- *Remove the dust in the room frequently*.

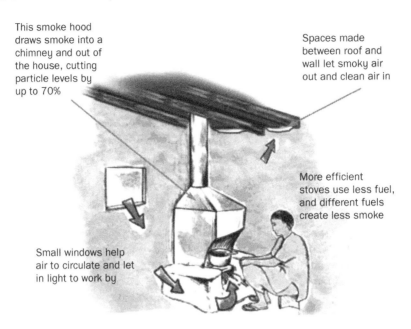

This smoke hood draws smoke into a chimney and out of the house, cutting particle levels by up to 70%

Spaces made between roof and wall let smoky air out and clean air in

More efficient stoves use less fuel, and different fuels create less smoke

Small windows help air to circulate and let in light to work by

Figure 6.3 Using technology to reduce household air pollution.

Source: http://www.itdg.org/images/smoke-diagram.gif

Healthy housing

In the previous section, we addressed biomass burning, and options for reducing its impact on health in low-income countries. We now go on to consider the fabric of houses and what can be done in this area to reduce impacts on health.

As a result of increasing recognition of the key role that housing plays in maintaining health, researchers and policy-makers are now beginning to develop international guidelines on 'healthy housing' to promote wellbeing through the design, construction, maintenance and location of homes (WHO 2010). In June 2009, the Surgeon General of the United States released a 'Call to Action to Promote Healthy Homes', stating that 'a healthy home is sited, designed, built, renovated, and maintained in ways that support the health of residents'.

Activity 6.4

Based on what you have learned in this chapter, what protections would you include in healthy housing guidelines? Try to list at least five protections, remembering that both the physical and social environment can influence the health of occupants.

Feedback

Here are some things you may have thought of:

- protection from weather and other environmental hazards;
- protection from fire;
- protection from air pollutants, chemicals and other toxic gases;
- protection against communicable disease;
- provision of essential services (such as clean water and sewerage);
- safe design and construction materials (to protect from injury);
- sustainability (particularly relating to the design and materials);
- energy efficiency (so that occupants can maintain adequate temperatures at reasonable cost and with reduced wider environmental impact);
- adequate space, privacy, comfort and security (reduces psychological stress).

A number of public health organizations have existing sets of principles for healthy housing. These include the US Centers for Disease Control and Protection (CDC) which has produced a *Healthy Housing Reference Manual*, reflecting the majority of areas above (CDC 2006). The WHO set out principles on healthy housing in 1989 and new guidelines on indoor air quality relating to household fuel combustion were published by WHO in 2014 (WHO 2014b), in response to the finding from the GBD study 2010 that air pollution from household fuel combustion is the most important global environmental health risk today (accounting for the highest burden of disease).

The new guidelines emphasize the importance of reducing fine particulate matter ($PM_{2.5}$) to gain most of the achievable health benefit, and highlight that most of the solid fuel interventions promoted in recent years have not even come close to achieving these levels when in everyday use. The recommendations for intervention focus particular attention on reducing emissions of pollutants (PM_{10}, CO, NO_x and others) as much as possible, while also recognizing the importance of adequate ventilation, and highlighting the need for community-wide action, as pollution from one house or other sources affects neighbours, and vice versa (WHO 2014b).

Another important consideration for healthy housing is sustainability and the reduction of greenhouse gas emissions associated with dwellings. This requires that housing is built of sustainable, non-polluting materials. Housing should be connected to amenities, non-polluting energy, water and sewerage, and located close to public transport, education and work opportunities, as well as green spaces (Wilkinson et al. 2007).

Building codes and standards

The development and implementation of building regulations are more upstream strategies for improving health in the indoor environment. Many countries have defined sets of minimum standards for buildings through legally-binding building codes, either at local or national level. In the European Union, a pan-European building code has now been implemented which supersedes all existing national codes (European Commission 2010). Such codes commonly define (among other things) appropriate materials for construction, requirements for energy provision and consumption, minimum and maximum room sizes and the provision of adequate emergency escape routes.

Summary

This chapter has summarized how housing can affect health. Health effects associated with household air pollution, overcrowding, indoor temperatures and damp were discussed. Improving the quality of housing, for example provision of adequate water and sanitation or adequate heating and cooling systems, has the potential to greatly improve the health of occupants. Household air pollution is a significant environmental health concern, especially in LMICs. The policy response to these challenges includes the development of guidelines on healthy housing; the continuing development of building standards.

References

Bates, M.N. et al. (2013) Acute lower respiratory infection in childhood and household fuel use in Bhaktapur, Nepal, *Environmental Health Perspectives,* 121: 637–42.

Bonjour, S. et al. (2013) Solid fuel use for household cooking: country and regional estimates for 1980–2010, *Environmental Health Perspectives,* 121: 784–90.

CDC (2006) *Healthy Housing Reference Manual.* Atlanta, GA: US Department of Health and Human Services.

EPA (2011) What are the trends in indoor air quality and their effects on human health?, http://cfpub.epa.gov/eroe/index.cfm?fuseaction=list.listBySubTopic&ch=46&s=343, accessed 12 June 2014.

European Commission (2010) EN Eurocodes, http://eurocodes.jrc.ec.europa.eu/.

Fisk, W.J., Lei-Gomez, Q. and Mendell, M.J. (2007) Meta-analyses of the associations of respiratory health effects with dampness and mold in homes, *Indoor Air,* 17(4): 284–96.

Green, G. and Gilbertson, J. (2008) *Warm Front, Better Health. Health impact evaluation of the Warm Front Scheme.* Sheffield: Centre for Regional, Economic and Social Research.

Hills, J. (2012) *Getting the Measure of Fuel Poverty: final report of the Fuel Poverty Review.* London: Centre for Analysis of Social Exclusion, LSE, Case Report 72, Crown copyright 2012, ISSN 1465-3001.

Jacobs, D.E., Wilson, J., Dixon, S.L., Smith, J. and Evens, A. (2009) The relationship of housing and population health: a 30-year retrospective analysis, *Environmental Health Perspectives,* 117(4): 597–604.

Kar, A. et al. (2012) Real-time assessment of black carbon pollution in Indian households due to traditional and improved biomass cookstoves, *Environmental Science & Technology*, 46(5): 2993–3000.

Krieger, J. and Higgins, D.L. (2002) Housing and health: time again for public health action, *American Journal of Public Health*, 92(5): 758–68.

Law, M.R., Morris, J.K. and Wald, N.J. (1997) Environmental tobacco smoke exposure and ischaemic heart disease: an evaluation of the evidence, *British Medical Journal*, 315(7114): 973–80.

Lee, P.N. and Forey, B.A. (2006) Environmental tobacco smoke exposure and risk of stroke in non-smokers: a review with meta-analysis, *Journal of Stroke and Cerebrovascular Diseases*, 15(5): 190–201.

Ministry of New and Renewable Energy (2009) *National Biomass Cookstoves Initiative*. India: Government of India.

Mølhave, L., Dueholm, S. and Jensen, L.K. (2004) Assessment of exposures and health risks related to formaldehyde emissions from furniture: a case study, *Indoor Air*, 5(2): 104–19.

Mudarri, D. and Fisk, W.J. (2007) Public health and economic impact of dampness and mold, *Indoor Air*, 17(3): 226–35.

National Cancer Institute (2011) Radon and cancer factsheet, http://www.cancer.gov/about-cancer/causes-prevention/risk/substances/radon/radon-fact-sheet, accessed 11 November 2015.

Office of the Deputy Prime Minister (2004) *The Impact of Overcrowding on Health & Education: a review of evidence and literature*. London: The Stationery Office.

Office of the Deputy Prime Minister (2006) *Housing Health and Safety Rating System. Operational guidance*. London: The Stationery Office.

Pope, C.A., III, Burnett, R.T., Thun, M.J. et al. (2002) Lung cancer, cardiopulmonary mortality, and long-term exposure to fine particulate air pollution, *Journal of the American Medical Association*, 287(9): 1132–41.

Smith, K.R. (2000) National burden of disease in India from indoor air pollution, *Proceedings of the National Academy of Sciences*, 97(24): 13286–93, http://www.pnas.org/content/97/24/13286.full, accessed 11 November 2015.

Smith, K.R. et al. (2011) Effect of reduction in household air pollution in childhood pneumonia in Guatemala (RESPIRE): a randomised control trial, *Lancet*, 378: 1717–26.

Smith, K.R. et al. (2014) Millions dead: how do we know and what does it mean? Methods used in the comparative risk assessment of household air pollution, *Annual Review of Public Health*, 35, http://www.annualreviews.org/doi/abs/10.1146/annurev-publhealth-032013-182356.

UK Parliament (2010) *UK Indoor Air Quality*, POSTNOTE 366, November, http://www.parliament.uk/business/publications/research/briefing-papers/POST-PN-366.

UN Foundations (2012) *Global Alliance for Clean Cookstoves 2010*, available at: http://www.cleancookstoves.org/the-alliance/, accessed 23 July 2013.

Vandentorren, S., Bretin, P., Zeghnoun, A. et al. (2006) August 2003 heat wave in France: risk factors for death of elderly people living at home, *European Journal of Public Health*, 19(6): 583–91.

WHO (2009) Estimated deaths & DALYs attributable to selected risk factors, http://www.who.int/indoorair/health_impacts/burden_national/en/index.html.

WHO (2010) Experts call for international guidelines on healthy housing, http://www.euro.who.int/en/health-topics/environment-and-health/pages/news/news/2010/11/experts-call-for-international-guidelines-on-healthy-housing, accessed 16 November 2015.

WHO (2014a) Burden of disease from household air pollution for 2012 – summary of results, http://www.who.int/phe/health_topics/outdoorair/databases/FINAL_HAP_AAP_BoD_24March2014.pdf, accessed 15 June 2014.

WHO (2014b) *WHO Guidelines for Indoor Air Quality: household fuel combustion*. Geneva: WHO, http://apps.who.int/iris/bitstream/10665/141496/1/9789241548885_eng.pdf?ua=1, accessed 11 November 2015.

Wilkinson, P. et al. (2004) Vulnerability to winter mortality in elderly people in Great Britain: population based study, *British Medical Journal*, 329(7467): 647.

Wilkinson, P., Smith, K.R., Joffe, M. and Haines, A. (2007) A global perspective on energy: health effects and injustices, *Lancet*, 370: 965–78.

Zhang, J. and Smith, K.R. (2007) Household air pollution from coal and biomass fuels in China: measurements, health impacts and interventions, *Environmental Health Perspectives*, 115: 848–55.

Outdoor air pollution and road transport

7

Cathryn Tonne and Noah Scovronick

Overview

Outdoor air pollution is a significant environmental health problem in high-, middle- and low-income countries. This chapter provides an overview of the sources of outdoor air pollution, the health effects of outdoor air pollutants and the methods used to quantify these health effects. It also discusses policy approaches to reduce harm to human health from outdoor air pollution. The chapter then focuses on road transport as an important source of outdoor air pollution. A broad overview of the health effects of road transport is provided as well as discussion of approaches to reduce the associated health burdens.

Learning objectives

At the end of this chapter you will be able to:

- describe the main outdoor air pollutants, their sources and their effects on human health
- describe the epidemiological methods for quantifying the health effects of outdoor air pollution
- evaluate a health impact assessment estimating the impact of air pollution on mortality and identify its key uncertainties
- describe the main health effects of road transport
- evaluate the trade-offs between health benefits and harms in transport policies

Key terms

Concentrations: The amount of a given pollutant found in the atmosphere, often expressed as parts per million or grams per cubic metre.

Emissions: Any form of pollution that is discharged into the environment.

Health impact assessment (HIA): A means of assessing the health impacts of policies, plans and projects in diverse economic sectors using quantitative, qualitative and participatory techniques.

Primary pollutant: A pollutant added directly to the atmosphere from natural or human ('anthropogenic') activity.

Secondary pollutant: A pollutant formed in the atmosphere when primary pollutants react in the atmosphere with other compounds.

Outdoor air pollution and public health

Air is considered to be polluted when it contains any extraneous constituent in sufficient quantities to adversely affect the environment or the health of people exposed to it. There is now a large body of evidence that suggests that negative health effects are linked to outdoor air pollution even at relatively low concentrations. Outdoor air pollution is a public health concern in urban areas worldwide (see Figure 7.1). It is estimated to account for 2 per cent of premature deaths globally: 1.9 per cent in low- and middle-income countries (LMICs) and 2.5 per cent in high-income countries (WHO 2009). Urban air pollution causes an estimated 8 per cent of deaths from lung cancer, 5 per cent of cardiopulmonary deaths and 3 per cent of deaths from respiratory infections (WHO 2009).

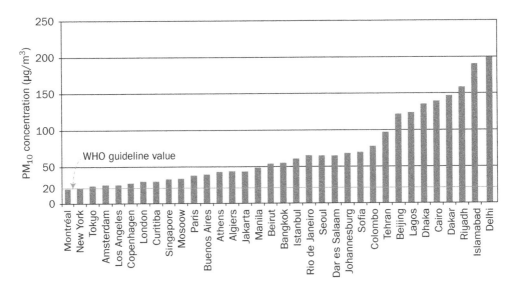

Figure 7.1 Average annual PM_{10} concentrations ($\mu g/m^3$) in a sample of large urban areas.
Source: WHO (2011).

Sources of air pollution

Outdoor air pollution originates from a number of different sources, which makes strategies for control difficult. The burning of fossil fuels for energy, and emissions from petrol- and diesel-powered vehicles are the dominant sources of anthropogenic outdoor air pollution. Natural sources of air pollution include forest fires, windblown dust and volcanic eruptions. Many sources of air pollution emit several different pollutants, giving rise to mixtures of pollutants in the air. Because the pollutants come from the same source, their concentrations are often highly correlated, presenting a challenge to the identification of the specific pollutant driving observed health effects.

 Activity 7.1

Think about where you live or work. What are the main local sources of outdoor air pollution in this area? When are people likely to come into contact with high levels of air pollution?

Feedback

The main sources of outdoor air pollution depend on the level of economic development and on air pollution management strategies, among other factors. In LMICs, the important sources are likely to be:

- agricultural and household solid fuel combustion (coal, wood, animal dung and crop residues which have no nutritional value, such as maize husks);
- transport;
- industry;
- fossil fuel-burning power stations.

This list is similar for high-income countries but there is less burning of solid fuels and a higher proportion of pollution tends to come from the transport sector.

Exposure to air pollution from the sources listed above depends heavily on their location relative to the population. For example, power plants and industrial sources are generally located in population-sparse areas, thereby reducing exposure. In urban areas, where road transport is a major source of pollution, exposures can be high, particularly for people inside vehicles and for those walking or cycling alongside such traffic. Furthermore, traffic-related air pollution is often higher within about 150 metres of major roads, exposing people who live near roads to more pollution. Household solid fuel combustion leads to very high indoor concentrations – covered in Chapter 6 – but it can also contribute to outdoor air pollution.

Types of air pollution

Air pollutants can be categorized based on their source, physical and chemical characteristics, or by how they are regulated. Table 7.1 lists several important air pollutants, with a list of their sources and health effects. Some of these pollutants are regulated in the European Union or have guidelines set by the WHO.

Air pollutants can also be categorized as primary or secondary pollutants. Primary pollutants are directly emitted by a source into the atmosphere. Secondary pollutants are formed in the atmosphere through physical and chemical processes (see Figure 7.2). Carbon monoxide (CO) is emitted directly from vehicle exhausts and is an example of a primary pollutant. This combines quickly in the outdoor air with oxygen to form carbon dioxide (CO_2) – a cause of climate change. CO_2 is also emitted directly from transport and other combustion processes. Thus, it is both a primary and a secondary pollutant. Ozone is not emitted directly in large amounts, but forms as a secondary pollutant through chemical reactions of other pollutants in the presence of sunlight. Primary pollutants that are subject to transformation to secondary pollutants are called *precursors* of that pollutant.

Some pollutants, like particulate matter (PM), are both directly emitted and also formed in the atmosphere from precursors. PM is a complex mixture of solid and liquid phase particles of varying composition and is often characterized by size. PM_{10} refers to particles 10 microns in diameter or less, $PM_{2.5}$ refers to particles 2.5 microns or less (also known as fine particles) and ultrafine particles are 0.1 microns or less in diameter. Mechanical grinding and windblown dust generate primary particles in the PM_{10} range, whereas secondary particles and many primary particles emitted by combustion are generally in the $PM_{2.5}$ size range. Particle size influences their deposition in the environment and in the respiratory system once they are inhaled. Smaller particles are of more interest for public health because they are deposited more deeply in the lungs.

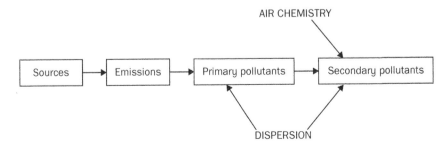

Figure 7.2 Dispersion and air chemistry in relation to pollutants.

Table 7.1 Summary of air pollutants, their sources, health effects and standards

Pollutant	Pollutant type	Key sources	Health effects*	Regulations/guidelines‡
Lead (Pb)	Primary	Leaded fuel, batteries, metal processing	Cancer, nervous system damage, cognitive disabilities	WHO Annual mean: 0.5 µg/m³ EU Annual: 0.5 µg/m³
Sulphur dioxide (SO_2)	Primary	Fossil fuel combustion (power plants or in the household), industrial boilers, oil refineries, decomposition of organic matter, sea spray, volcanic eruptions	Respiratory symptoms Precursor to PM sulphate	WHO 10-minute mean: 500 µg/m³ 24-hour mean: 20 µg/m³ EU 1-hour mean: 350 µg/m³ 24-hour mean: 125 µg/m³
Carbon monoxide (CO)	Primary	Fossil fuel combustion, forest fires, natural	Fatigue, headache, neurological damage, dizziness	WHO 15-minute mean: 100,000 µg/m³ 30-minute mean: 60,000 µg/m³ 1-hour mean: 30,000 µg/m³ 8-hour mean: 10,000 µg/m³ EU Maximum daily 8-hour mean: 10,000 µg/m³
Particulate matter ($PM_{2.5}$, PM_{10})	Primary and secondary	Fossil fuel combustion, biomass burning, natural sources such as pollen, conversion of $NO_x/SO_x/$ VOCs, dust storms, forest fires, dirt roads	Respiratory symptoms, exacerbation of respiratory and cardiovascular disease, mortality	WHO $PM_{2.5}$: Annual mean: 10 µg/m³ 24-hour mean: 25 µg/m³ PM_{10}: Annual mean: 20 µg/m³ 24-hour mean 50 µg/m³ EU $PM_{2.5}$: Annual mean: 25 µg/m³ mean 3-year mean: 20 µg/m³ ** PM_{10}: 24-hour mean: 50 µg/m³ Annual mean: 40 µg/m³

Table 7.1 Summary of air pollutants, their sources, health effects and standards (Continued)

Pollutant	Pollutant type	Key sources	Health effects*	Regulations/guidelines‡
Nitrogen oxides (NO_x, NO_2)	Primary and secondary	Fossil fuel combustion, kerosene heaters, biological processes in soil, lightning	Respiratory symptoms and infection Ozone precursor Contributes to PM nitrate	For NO_2: WHO 1-hour mean: 200 µg/ Annual mean: 40 µg/m^3 EU 1-hour mean: 200 µg/m^3 Annual mean: 40 µg/m^3
Tropospheric ozone (O_3)	Secondary	Formed from chemical reactions of precursors (VOCs and NOx) in the presence of sunlight	Respiratory symptoms, eye irritation, bronchoconstriction, mortality	WHO 8-hour mean: 100 µg/m^3 EU Maximum daily 8-hour mean: 120 µg/m^3
'Toxic pollutants' (e.g. asbestos, mercury, dioxins, some VOCs)†	Primary and secondary	Industrial processes, solvents, paint thinners, fuel	Cancer, reproductive effects, neurological damage, respiratory effects	Regulations/guidelines for specific compounds
Volatile organic compounds (VOCs)	Primary and secondary	Solvents, glues, smoking, fuel combustion, vegetation, forest fires	Dependent on the compound Irritation of respiratory tract, nausea, cancer Ozone precursor PM precursors	Regulations/guidelines for specific compounds
Biological pollutants	Primary	Vegetation, animals Heating/cooling systems can encourage production	Allergic reactions, respiratory symptoms, fatigue, asthma	

Notes

* List of sources and health effects is not exhaustive.

‡ Some values are target values – will only become legally binding limits in the future. A certain number of exceedences are permitted for some pollutants.

** Average exposure indicator determined using selected monitoring stations in larger urban areas to best assess general population exposure to $PM_{2.5}$.

† Lead is also often referred to as a toxic pollutant, although it is treated separately in this table.

Source: Adapted from Bell and Samet (2005).

Factors influencing pollution concentrations

Air pollution is often measured as the mass of a pollutant per volume of air, which is a concentration. Air pollution concentrations in a particular location depend on many factors, including activity from local emission sources, the transport of pollution from distant sources to the area where the concentration is being measured ('long-range' air pollution), weather and land patterns. Temperature, wind speed and direction, amount of sunlight, and level of precipitation are important weather-related factors influencing concentrations. Consequently, many pollutants show considerable variability over seasons and time of day.

Studying the health effects of air pollutants

In order to understand the impact of air pollution on health, a variety of approaches are used including:

- laboratory studies on humans and animal models;
- epidemiological (population) studies including time series and cohort studies.

Laboratory studies use small numbers of subjects, but allow a detailed examination of the physiological and toxicological effects of controlled levels of exposure to help establish the biological mechanism of health effects.

Epidemiological studies involve larger numbers of people and assess the association between pollutants and health in the general environment at the population level. Studies of the acute health effects of short-term exposures generally compare the daily fluctuations in exposures with those in health using time-series (or case-crossover) analyses. Studies of the health effects of exposures over a longer term compare the occurrence of disease over several years across individuals or communities with varying levels of exposure. A brief overview of the main types of epidemiological studies used to investigate the health effects of air pollution follows.

Short-term exposure and health

Daily time-series designs have been used to analyse the associations between short-term (acute) exposure to air pollution and counts of mortality or hospital admissions. These studies:

- allow comparison of daily changes in pollution with those in health;
- require adjustment for time-varying health risk factors, including long-term trends, season, day of week, temperature, influenza and other respiratory infections;

- provide estimates only of acute effects reflecting exacerbation of disease and precipitation of deaths, which may have been brought forward only by a few weeks, so cannot be used to estimate how much lives have been shortened.

Such time-series studies suggest that on days of high pollution, deaths, hospital admissions and general practice consultations may rise by at most a few per cent compared with days of low pollution. There is also evidence that short-term increases in exposure to air pollution are associated with increased rates of cardiac arrhythmia and levels of inflammation (Rückerl et al. 2011). The evidence is especially strong for a relationship between PM (PM_{10} and $PM_{2.5}$) and deaths from all cardiovascular causes. Positive associations between PM_{10} and daily all-cause and cardiovascular mortality have been observed in large multi-city time-series studies in Europe – all-cause: 0.6 per cent per 10 µg/m³ (95 per cent confidence interval 0.4, 0.8 per cent) (Katsouyanni et al. 2001) – and the USA – all-cause: 0.5 per cent per 10 µg/m³ (95 per cent CI 0.1, 0.9 per cent) (Samet et al. 2000). Similar results have been observed in several different countries.

Long-term exposure and health

Health effects arising from exposures over the longer term may come about through a different mechanism than for acute effects (Brook et al. 2010). To study the long-term impact of air pollution, cohort or cross-sectional studies are undertaken to compare the incidence or prevalence of disease in populations exposed to different long-term average levels of pollution. These studies can provide information on the amount of life lost due to exposure, as well as occurrence of mortality, but need to take account of the potentially strong confounding effects of socioeconomic circumstances, smoking and other behavioural factors, which tend to differ across communities. In common with all population-based studies, there are difficulties in measuring exposure, especially over long periods of time. The health changes associated with longer-term exposure to air pollution have generally been found to be larger than those from shorter-term exposure.

A number of large cohort studies have shown that elevated levels of $PM_{2.5}$ were associated with all-cause and cardio-respiratory mortality and cardiovascular morbidity (Pope et al. 2002; Brook et al. 2010). It has been estimated that people living in the most polluted US cities would have lost between 1.8 and 3.1 years of life because of exposure to chronic air pollution (Pope et al. 2009).

Large cohort studies are expensive and logistically difficult to conduct. Consequently, nearly all of the studies of long-term exposure to outdoor air pollution have been carried out in high-income countries. There is a need for such studies in rapidly developing countries that are experiencing increasing urbanization and vehicle use. Findings from high-income countries may not be generalizable to these settings because of differences in air pollution mixtures, overall levels of exposure (concentrations are generally substantially higher than those observed in high-income settings) and susceptibility.

Determining the exact level of exposure of an individual level is, however, complicated. Epidemiological studies tend to use either ambient air pollution monitors or modelled pollutant concentrations to assign exposure, but these methods cannot fully account for people moving between different areas and between indoor and outdoor environments. More detailed monitoring (e.g. personal, micro-environmental) is usually not feasible for large population studies or long periods of time.

 Activity 7.2

How might you use epidemiological evidence to estimate the burden of premature mortality (numbers of excess deaths) due to exposure to particles from anthropogenic sources in your country?

Feedback

Health impact assessment is a useful tool for quantifying this sort of burden. In order to make a rough estimate of the burden you will need several pieces of information. The following example is based on $PM_{2.5}$ in the UK, but the approach could be used in other countries.

What is the population exposure to $PM_{2.5}$ from anthropogenic sources?

The population-weighted average $PM_{2.5}$ levels in the UK have been previously estimated by combining a map of modelled $PM_{2.5}$ for every 1 km^2 and multiplying it by the proportion of the total population who live in that square kilometre (Committee on the Medical Effects of Air Pollutants 2010). For the UK, the population weighted average in 2008 was estimated to be 10.4 µg/m^3. However, only about 86 per cent of that $PM_{2.5}$ is from anthropogenic sources – the remainder is of natural origin. This is known from 'source apportionment' studies. We therefore assume the population exposure to anthropogenic $PM_{2.5}$ is:

$$0.86*10.4 \text{ µg/m}^3 = 8.9 \text{ µg/m}^3$$

How can we relate this to health?

This is where the epidemiological evidence comes in. Specifically, we use information from epidemiological studies that have been conducted elsewhere and apply the findings to our study population. As mentioned earlier, the mortality effects of long-term exposure to $PM_{2.5}$ are generally larger than the effects of short-term exposure, so time-series studies underestimate the total burden. We therefore would select a cohort study of long-term exposure to $PM_{2.5}$ as the basis of our exposure-response estimate. The American Cancer Society study is often used for this purpose because it is a large study and the findings have been carefully checked by external investigators. In this study, the relative risk (RR) of death was 1.06 (i.e. 6 per cent) for a $10 \, \mu g/m^3$ increase in $PM_{2.5}$ based on a log-linear model (Pope et al. 2002).

First we need to rescale this estimate to get the RR for a $8.9 \, \mu g/m^3$ change in $PM_{2.5}$.

Although strictly we should take the logarithm of 1.06, to a good approximation we can rescale the 6 per cent:

> % increase in RR for an $8.9 \, \mu g/m^3 = 6*8.9/10 = 5.3\%$,
> or RR = 1.05 (rounding)

For those interested in the mathematically correct sequence, as the RR was based on a log-linear model – in other words, the natural log (ln) of the RR is linearly associated with $PM_{2.5}$, then

RR for 10 unit change = exp(b*10) = 1.06 where b is the natural log RR for a 1 unit change in $PM_{2.5}$.

> b*10 = ln(1.06)
> b = ln(1.06)/10 = 0.0058

> The RR for a 1 unit change is then exp(0.0058) = 1.0058
> And the RR for an $8.9 \, \mu g/m^3$ change is exp(0.0058*8.9) = 1.05

How do we estimate the attributable burden?

First we calculate the attributable fraction (AF) of deaths due to anthropogenic exposure using the following formula:

> AF = (RR – 1)/RR
> AF = (1.05 – 1)/1.05 = 0.05 (rounded)

This tells us the *proportion* of disease burden among the exposed that can be attributed to exposure.

A rough estimate of the total number of deaths in the UK per year is 600,000. We can therefore estimate that 600,000 x 0.05 or about 30,000 deaths per year would have been brought forward in time because of exposure to anthropogenic pollution if they had experienced the 2008 concentrations over a long period. (The term 'brought forward' is used because these people will die eventually – the effect of the air pollution is to shorten their lives.) Further discussion of this calculation is in Public Health England (2014).

What should you keep in mind?

This simple calculation sets aside several complexities and makes many assumptions, for example:

1 The relationship between $PM_{2.5}$ and death is causal.
2 The relationship between exposure and risk of death (strictly log risk) is linear – we assumed that the relationship was a straight line, but the exposure-response curve could take a non-linear shape (Burnett et al. 2014).
3 This calculation does not tell us how much earlier the deaths are occurring because of air pollution exposure. More sophisticated calculations, which are beyond the scope of this book, estimate the number of months or years of life that are lost in a population due to exposure. For example, it has been estimated that, in the UK, eliminating all exposure to anthropogenic $PM_{2.5}$ would increase life expectancy by an average of six months (Committee on the Medical Effects of Air Pollutants 2010).

As illustrated in the calculations above, an important feature of health effects from air pollution, and indeed many environmental exposures, is that increases in death or disability of only a few per cent can lead to large numbers of excess deaths or disease due to the size of the population exposed.

Policy approaches to outdoor air pollution

Several policy approaches to controlling air pollution exist, including setting ambient air quality standards, emission standards, technological controls and those implemented through market-based and voluntary approaches.

Air quality standards have been established in the USA, Europe and many other countries on the basis of protecting human health. The WHO also provides guidelines for certain pollutants. These standards set limits on concentrations of specific pollutants in outdoor air (refer back to Table 7.1). They apply over different averaging times which relate to whether the associated health effects are linked to short-term elevations in concentrations or their long-term average (or both). Although these standards are based on health, they may not always adequately protect individuals who are particularly susceptible (e.g. elderly people, children, those with pre-existing disease).

Emission standards are used to control specific sources by limiting the amount of a specific pollutant that can be emitted from that source, and are applied to stationary sources like power plants as well as mobile sources. Examples of implementation include fuel economy standards for vehicles (indirect effect on emissions including CO_2), or pollution control devices (e.g. exhaust catalysts on motor vehicles). Changes in fuel composition such as the removal of lead from gasoline (petrol) in most countries have also contributed to important reductions in toxic emissions. The use of liquid biofuels is another potential intervention, although the overall health impacts are still uncertain (see Activity 7.3).

Market-based approaches to air pollution control are increasingly used alongside other control policies. An example of a market-based approach is emissions trading programmes, in which a cap on the total amount of emissions of a specific pollutant is set and emitters trade permits in an open market. Emissions trading is most commonly discussed for carbon, but also other pollutants such as NOx. This approach aims to make lower emissions financially advantageous, although critics raise concerns about how the emissions threshold is determined (what level is acceptable and whether the required data are available), the procedure for allocating the permits (e.g. if permits are freely allocated or auctioned), and also question the ability of governments to enforce the trading schemes.

An additional approach to protect public health is to implement air pollution alert systems that warn susceptible individuals on high air pollution days so that they may modify their behaviour (e.g. stay indoors, delay physical activity) on that day to reduce their personal exposure.

Road transport and health

Worldwide energy use from the transport sector has risen steadily (between 2–2.5 per cent per year) since the early 1970s (IEA 2009). This growth has been largely in parallel with growth in global economic activity and is projected to continue increasing in the future. The largest growth in absolute terms has been in passenger vehicles and trucks. Trends since 2000 indicate that the largest growth in road transport has been in LMICs, where there has been larger population and economic growth compared to high-income countries (IEA 2009).

While there have been enormous societal benefits of increased road transport, including increased access to employment and educational opportunities and improved distribution of food, there have also been substantial costs to the environment and public health. In the remainder of this chapter, we provide an overview of the primary negative health impacts of road transport and measures that can be taken to reduce these impacts.

Traffic-related air pollution

As discussed earlier in the chapter, road transport is an important source of many air pollutants including PM, nitrogen oxides (NO_x), volatile organic compounds and carbon monoxide. For example, in Greater London, road transport is estimated to contribute 60 per cent of PM_{10}, 30 per cent of NO_x and 50 per cent of CO emissions (GLA 2008). While there is a large body of evidence investigating the link between exposure to air pollution from all sources combined, less evidence is available specifically regarding air pollution from traffic sources. However, this evidence base is growing rapidly. Exposures to traffic-related air pollution are typically measured based on proximity to roads, or modelled based on information on the location and emissions from sources. The evidence that specifically traffic-related air pollution causes exacerbation of symptoms among asthmatic children is strong (HEI 2009). The evidence for causation is less strong for mortality, cardiovasuclar morbidity, asthma incidence in children and respiratory symptoms in adults, while it is insufficient regarding the relationship with other health outcomes including adverse birth outcomes and cancer (HEI 2009). In the absence of sufficient evidence for pollution from traffic alone, estimates of the impact of traffic pollution on health use the relative risks derived from studies of total air pollution.

 Activity 7.3

Liquid biofuels, which are fuels derived from plant biomass, are currently one of the few available alternatives to fossil fuels for use in motor vehicle transport. Studies have found that liquid biofuels often produce fewer tailpipe PM_{10} emissions when compared to fossil fuels (Niven 2005; McCormick 2007). However, this finding does not necessarily equate to reduced air pollution-related health burdens. What other factors do you think should be considered when assessing the impacts on air quality and hence on health of a change in vehicle fuel?

Feedback

Other important factors you might have considered include:

- *The size of the PM emissions:* although PM_{10} is associated with ill-health, attention is increasingly focused on fine particles ($PM_{2.5}$). Reduced PM_{10} emissions does not always mean reduced $PM_{2.5}$ emissions, although the two are usually strongly correlated.
- *The composition of PM:* PM is a heterogeneous mix of particles. Some components of PM may be more toxic than others and the composition of PM emissions depends partly on the fuel type used.
- *Other pollutants:* PM is not the only pollutant of concern with regard to public health; other pollutants such as ozone are also associated with negative health effects. Combustion of liquid biofuels releases ozone precursors and may increase the formation of ground-level ozone (Jacobson 2007). Different transport fuels may therefore reduce emissions of some health-relevant air pollutants, but increase others.
- *Emissions at other stages in the biofuel life-cycle:* although liquid biofuels often show reduced exhaust emissions, emissions during production and distribution can be high.

Biofuels are discussed in more detail in Chapter 11.

Road traffic injuries

Road traffic crashes cause 1.3 million deaths per year globally and approximately 20–50 million additional people suffer non-fatal injuries. Road traffic accidents are the leading cause of death among young people (aged 15–29) and the burden is particularly high in LMICs where over 90 per cent of global traffic fatalities occur. Within high-income countries, people living in lower socioeconomic conditions are more likely to be involved in road traffic accidents compared to others who are better off (WHO 2012).

If historical trends continue, it is projected that traffic fatalities will increase from 2000 to 2020 by 66 per cent globally, with large disparities (health inequalities) between countries (see Figure 7.3). However, these projections are based on limited data, particularly in low-income countries, which are likely to have the highest fatality rates.

The harm from road transport can be viewed as the product of (1) potentially risky conditions, (2) the probability of a crash in those conditions, and (3) the consequence of the crash (e.g. fatality, injury) (Sivak and Tsimhoni 2008). Measures to promote road safety can target any of these three dimensions. Several features in road design aim to reduce harm primarily for vehicle occupants, but may also benefit other vulnerable road users like pedestrians and cyclists. Seatbelts have been an important safety measure in reducing the consequences for occupants in the event of a crash; seatbelts are estimated to reduce the risk of serious and fatal injuries by 40 and 65 per cent repectively (Ameratunga et al. 2006).

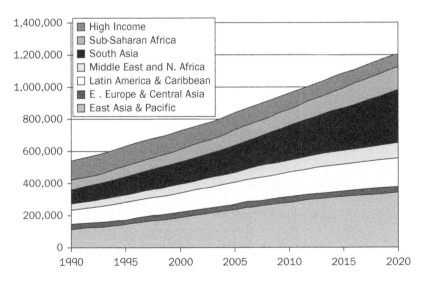

Figure 7.3 Global traffic fatalities, adjusted for under-reporting, 1990–2020.
Source: Koptis et al. (2005).

Physical inactivity

Globally, physical inactivity is estimated to cause 6–10 per cent of major non-communicable diseases, including coronary heart disease, type 2 diabetes, and breast and colon cancers; it also contributes to premature mortality (Lee et al. 2012). Physical inactivity is also a risk factor for over-weight and obesity, which together affect over a billion people worldwide and are the fifth leading risk for global deaths (WHO 2009).

Widespread motorization has important implications for physical activity by replacing active forms of transportation such as walking and cycling with sedentary forms. Increased reliance on motorized transport over the past decades in high-income countries is likely to have played a role in increasing rates of physical inactivity.

There is good evidence that commuter walking and cycling are beneficial for reducing all-cause mortality (Hallal et al. 2012). Active commuting among children has been associated with reduced body-mass index and reduced cardiovascular risk factors (Hallal et al. 2012). The benefits of physical activity and how this can be facilitated by appropriate urban planning are discussed in Chapter 9. These benefits should be considered against the risks of injury from road traffic accidents and increased exposure to air pollution from individuals participating in walking and cycling. The relative trade-offs in terms of health risks are likely to depend on local contexts.

Noise

Excessive noise, or unwanted sound, is harmful for health and interferes with people's daily activities at home, work and school. In many urban areas, road transport is a major source of environmental noise as well as air pollution. Noise from road transport depends on the distance from source, traffic volumes and vehicle mix as well as the surrounding topography (e.g. building heights) of an area. Environmental noise has been associated with cardiovascular disease (Selander et al. 2009; Gan et al. 2012); cognitive impairment in children (WHO Europe 2011); disruption of sleep and annoyance (Pirrera et al. 2010). Noise from road transport may be tackled by reducing the amount of noise produced per vehicle, reducing the number or speed of vehicles in an area, constructing sound barriers, or siting of major roadways away from residences and workplaces.

Activity 7.4

Imagine the city of Delhi, India, in the year 2030 under the following scenarios:

1 Business as usual: projection of existing trends in population and increasing car use, with some increase in rail use.

2 Low emission motor vehicles: mandatory lower emission motor vehicles and use of alternative fuels.
3 Increased active travel: reversal of present trends in car use and reductions in motorcycle use; large increases in walking, cycling, and rail use

What would be the implications of each scenario for health? Which health outcomes would you consider? Which impacts on health would you expect to be the largest?

Feedback

The impacts of these three scenarios on health and carbon dioxide (CO_2) emissions were modelled by Woodcock and colleagues (Woodcock et al. 2009). They modelled the impact of: 1) physical activity on several health outcomes including heart disease, stroke, diabetes and some cancers; 2) $PM_{2.5}$ on mortality from cardio-respiratory disease and lung cancer in adults and acute respiratory infections in children; and 3) motor vehicle traffic on the number of pedestrians and cyclists injured in road accidents.

The following table summarizes results from this modelling including the PM and CO_2 emissions per person per year for each scenario. The years of life gained per million population over a one-year period are presented for each scenario compared to business as usual.

Table 7.2 Differing transport scenarios and estimated impacts on health

Scenario	$PM_{2.5}$ concentration ($\mu g/m^3$)	CO_2 emissions per person-year (tonnes)	Years of life gained from physical activity	Years of life gained from air pollution	Years of life gained from avoided road traffic crashes
Business as usual	90	0.75	–	–	–
Low emission motor vehicles	79	0.66	0	1696	0
Increased active travel	76	0.40	6040	2240	2809

These results indicate that switching to low emitting vehicles generated some health gains through lower air pollution exposures. Much larger health gains were achieved through the active travel scenario, partly due to lower air pollution exposures, but also through increased physical activity and reduced road traffic crashes. The largest benefits in the increased active travel scenario were from increased physical activity, particularly through reduction in the prevalence of heart disease, stroke and diabetes.

Summary

This chapter has provided broad overviews of the related, but distinct, topics of outdoor air pollution and road transport in relation to human health. Several outdoor air pollutants are relevant for human health and these are generated from a range of sources. Time-series and cohort studies are the primary epidemiological study designs that have given rise to the now large body of evidence regarding the health effects of outdoor air pollution. There are a number of strategies available to reduce outdoor air pollution, including implementing air quality and emission standards, emission trading schemes, and encouraging the use of cleaner technologies, among others. Road transport is not only an important source of human exposure to air pollution but also presents a risk of injury and has implications for health through reduced physical activity.

References

Ameratunga, S., Hijar, M. and Norton, R. (2006) Road-traffic injuries: confronting disparities to address a global-health problem, *Lancet*, 367: 1533–40.

Bell, M.L. and Samet, J.M. (2005) Air pollution, in H. Frumkin (ed.) *Environmental Health: from global to local*, pp. 331–61. San Francisco: Jossey-Bass.

Brook, R.D., Rajagopalan, S., Pope, C.A. et al. (2010) Particulate matter air pollution and cardiovascular disease. An update to the scientific statement from the American Heart Association, *Circulation*, 121: 2331–78.

Burnett, R.T., Arden Pope III, C., Olives, C., et al. (2014) An Integrated Risk Function for Estimating the Global Burden of Disease Attributable to Ambient Fine Particulate Matter Exposure. EHP.

Committee on the Medical Effects of Air Pollutants (2010) *The Mortality Effects of Long-term Exposure to Particulate Air Pollution in the United Kingdom*, https://www.gov.uk/government/publications/comeap-mortality-effects-of-long-term-exposure-to-particulate-air-pollution-in-the-uk.

Gan, W.Q., Davies, H.W., Koehoorn, M. and Brauer, M. (2012) Association of long-term exposure to community noise and traffic-related air pollution with coronary heart disease mortality, *American Journal of Epidemiology*, 175: 898–906.

GLA (Greater London Authority) (2008) *London Atmospheric Emissions Inventory 2004 Report*. London: Greater London Authority.

Hallal, P.C., Andersen, L.B., Bull, F.C., Guthold, R., Haskell, W. and Ekelund, U. (2012) Global physical activity levels: surveillance progress, pitfalls, and prospects, *Lancet*, 380: 247–57.

HEI (Health Effects Institute) (2009) *Traffic-Related Air Pollution: a critical review of the literature on emissions, exposures, and health effects*. Boston, MA: Health Effects Institute.

IEA (International Energy Agency) (2009) *Transport, Energy, and CO₂*. Paris: IEA.

Jacobson, M. (2007) Effects of ethanol (E85) versus gasoline vehicles on cancer and mortality in the United States, *Environmental Science and Technology*, 41: 4150–7.

Katsouyanni, K., Touloumi, G., Samoli, E. et al. (2001) Confounding and effect modification in the short-term effects of ambient particles on total mortality: results from 29 European cities within the APHEA2 Project, *Epidemiology*, 12: 521–31.

Kopits, E. and Cropper, M. (2005) Traffic fatalities and economic growth, *Accident Analysis and Prevention*, 37(1): 169–78.

Lee, I-M., Shiroma, E.J., Lobelo, F., Puska, P., Blair, S.N. and Katzmarzyk, P.T. (2012) Effect of physical inactivity on major non-communicable diseases worldwide: an analysis of burden of disease and life expectancy, *Lancet*, 380: 219–29.

McCormick, R.L. (2007) The impact of biodiesel on pollutant emissions and public health, *Inhalation Toxicology*, 19: 1033–9.

Niven, R. (2005) Ethanol in gasoline: environmental impacts and sustainability review article, *Renewable and Sustainable Energy Reviews*, 9: 535–55.

Pirrera, S., Valck, E. De and Cluydts, R. (2010) Nocturnal road traffic noise: a review on its assessment and consequences on sleep and health, *Environment International*, 36: 492–8.

Pope, C.A. III et al. (2002) Lung cancer, cardiopulmonary mortality, and long-term exposure to fine particulate air pollution, *Journal of the American Medical Association*, 287: 1132–41.

Pope, C.A. III, Ezzati, M. and Dockery, D.W. (2009) Fine-particulate matter air pollution and life expectancy in the United States, *New England Journal of Medicine*, 360(4): 376–86.

Public Health England (2014) PHE-CRCE-010: estimating local mortality burdens associated with particulate air pollution, https://www.gov.uk/government/publications/estimating-local-mortality-burdens-associated-with-particulate-air-pollution.

Rückerl, R., Schneider, A., Breitner, S., Cyrys, J. and Peters, A. (2011) Health effects of particulate air pollution: a review of epidemiological evidence, *Inhalation Toxicology*, 23: 555–92.

Samet, J.M., Dominici, F., Curriero, F.C., Coursac, I. and Zeger, S.L. (2000) Fine particulate air pollution and mortality in 20 U.S. cities, 1987–1994, *New England Journal of Medicine*, 343: 1742–9.

Selander, J. et al. (2009) Long-term exposure to road traffic noise and myocardial infarction, *Epidemiology*, 20: 272–9.

Sivak, M. and Tsimhoni, O. (2008) Improving traffic safety: conceptual considerations for successful action, *Journal of Safety Research*, 39: 453–7.

WHO (2009) *Global Health Risks: mortality and burden of disease attributable to selected major risks*. Geneva: WHO.

WHO (2011) Database: outdoor air pollution in cities, http://www.who.int/phe/health_topics/outdoorair/databases/cities-2011/en/, accessed 3 May 2016.

WHO (2012) Road traffic injuries, http://www.who.int/mediacentre/factsheets/fs358/en/index.html#.

WHO Europe (2011) *Burden of Disease from Environmental Noise*. Geneva: WHO.

Woodcock, J., Edwards, P., Tonne, C. et al. (2009) Public health benefits of strategies to reduce greenhouse-gas emissions: urban land transport, *Lancet*, 374: 1930–43.

Waste

Araceli Busby

8

Overview

Waste is a key issue for environmental sustainability, not only because of the increasing volumes of waste being produced globally but also as a result of changing waste composition due to the production, consumption and inclusion in waste streams of more and more complex products. This chapter gives a brief overview of definitions of different kinds of waste, sources of waste and current options for managing waste. It then looks at the evidence for the health effects associated with different waste disposal options.

Learning objectives

By the end of this chapter you will be able to:

- summarize the main types of waste and waste disposal strategies
- describe the routes of human exposure to waste
- evaluate the evidence for the health impacts of different waste disposal strategies
- understand the key global issues in waste management

Key terms

Energy from waste (also termed incineration):   The method of solid waste disposal in which waste is burned at high temperatures in incinerator plants.

Hazardous waste: Waste which has properties that make it capable of harming human health.

Landfill: The burying of waste in the ground. Such disposal methods range from unmanaged burial through to highly technical engineered constructions with leachate and gas disposal systems.

Municipal waste: Waste generated by households and wastes of a similar nature generated by commercial establishments and from public places for which the local government administration usually has collection/disposal responsibility.

Special waste: A term sometimes used to encompass any waste that is neither municipal nor hazardous but is still governed by specific laws and regulations (e.g. medical waste, construction debris, mining waste, electrical goods and their components, batteries, etc.).

Introduction to waste and waste management

Waste production impacts on our environment in a variety of ways which can affect human health and quality of life. These include the visual impact of litter (dumping of waste in non-designated locations) and waste management facilities; air pollution and other pollutants from decomposing or incinerated waste; and greenhouse gas emissions. Other environmental impacts include energy use for transport and waste management; water pollution from leachate and other unregulated discharges; and contamination of land through landfilling.

In order to minimize the health and environmental impacts of waste, strategies to manage waste are necessary. As global population has increased and countries undergo economic development, the quantity and character of waste produced has changed. Industrialization has resulted in a waste stream which is complex and varied, requiring more diverse disposal methods. Key drivers in waste management (see Table 8.1) have resulted in

Table 8.1 Key drivers in the development of waste management

Key driver	Effect on policy
Public health	Concerns about health risks lead to policy development.
Environmental protection	Focus has shifted from eliminating uncontrolled disposal to systematic increasing of technical standards.
Climate change	Policies to control climate change (mitigation) need to address greenhouse gas emissions from waste.
The resource value of waste	People making a living from discarded materials remains important in low-income countries today.
Institutional and responsibility issues	Derived from the impact of the other drivers on government and business strategy.
Public awareness	Acts as a key driver for institutional strategic and legislative change.

Source: After Wilson (2007). See also UNEP (2010), Contreras et al. (2010), Zaman (2013)

considerable technological development and subsequent changes in waste management practices.

In the UK the impact of waste management on public health was a concern as early as 1839, when the link between sanitation and infectious disease prompted the first Public Health Act. The second Public Health Act in 1948 placed formal responsibility on local authorities for municipal waste collection. However, until the 1970s solid waste disposal continued to be relatively uncontrolled and consisted largely of dumping or burning. In the 1970s a number of high-profile stories of health effects associated with illegal hazardous waste dumps (e.g. Love Canal – see Beck 1979), as well as the emergence of environmental protection as a key driver, put waste disposal more firmly on the political agenda. Since the 1970s technological advances in high-income countries have changed waste management practices considerably. In low- and middle-income countries (LMICs), waste management may be limited by lack of resources or access to technology.

What is waste?

Waste may be defined broadly as any material, substance or product that the owner no longer wants at a given place and time. Such a judgement may be subjective and vary over time and according to economic necessity or technological advancement.

 Activity 8.1

In terms of the classification of waste, can you think of different ways in which waste could be classified or grouped? What do you think are the advantages of classifying waste by different methods?

Feedback

Waste can be classified in a variety of ways:

- by source;
- by physical form and biochemical material composition;
- by the management practices and legislative controls surrounding its disposal.

Different classification methods may each have particular advantages and disadvantages.

- *By source*: this gives only a very broad indication of the waste form and composition (e.g. domestic waste may have a wide variety of components); however, it is a valuable tool in developing and monitoring waste management policy. For example, the impact of a 'pay-as-you-throw' household waste charge on the quantity of domestic waste produced.

- *By composition*: this may be a valuable tool for decision-making about the most appropriate disposal options. For example, analysis of the composition of mobile phones, which contain minute amounts of different precious metals, suggests recycling has the potential to recover valuable resources.
- *By management practices and regulatory frameworks*: this provides information about changing practices and regulatory compliance, although it is less useful for evaluating how waste generation may be influenced.

Waste sources

Waste is produced from a wide variety of domestic and industrial sources. Construction and mining generate the greatest quantity of waste by weight (see Figure 8.1). Other sources produce waste which is extremely heterogeneous with constituents from many different sources (e.g. packaging and electronic goods). Household waste accounts for less than 10 per cent of all waste generated although it is the focus of much public concern.

Waste composition

The composition of waste from different sources (particularly municipal waste) varies from country to country and over time. For example, East Asia and the Pacific regions have a far higher proportion of organic waste compared with

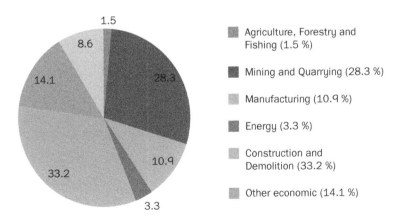

Figure 8.1 Waste generation in the EU-28 by economic activity 2010 (percentage by 1,000 tons).

Source: Adapted from Hartmut Schrör (2011).

OECD countries. As a country's affluence increases, organic and inert wastes generally decrease in relative terms, while paper and plastics increase.

Certain wastes that have properties that make them capable of harming human health or the environment are consequently defined as 'hazardous'. Characteristics which define hazard potential include ignitability, corrosiveness, reactivity and toxicity, and what precisely constitutes hazardous waste is often defined by legislation (see below).

Waste policy and legislation

Waste is commonly classified according to the rules and regulations governing its management and these may vary considerably around the world. While there are a number of international laws governing, for example, the transport of wastes, differences in individual countries' management and legislation have resulted in some countries transporting waste overseas to take advantage of less stringent laws and hence cheaper disposal costs. Differences in the legislative definition of hazardous waste in particular has in the past resulted in a thriving industry in the shipment of hazardous waste from industrialized countries to less well developed countries, where there is less legislation and regulation governing disposal. This is discussed further later in this chapter in the section on global issues.

How much waste do we produce?

The World Bank estimates that, worldwide, 1.3 billion tons of municipal solid waste are produced each year and forecasts a rise to 2.2 billion tons by 2025 (Hoornweg and Bhada-Tata 2012). Waste is also increasing in complexity and variety as well as overall quantity (Scheinberg et al. 2010). Comparison of the type and quantity of waste produced by different countries or regions is complicated by the unreliability of the data, particularly from LMICs, and also due to differences in waste classification (Hoornweg and Bhada-Tata 2012). For example, OECD statistics report household waste quantities, whereas US statistics report municipal waste quantities (which, as well as households, includes commercial properties, offices, etc.).

High-income countries produce much more waste per capita than low- and middle-income countries (LMICs). For example, the USA, with less than 5 per cent of the world's population, produces a third of the global quantity of solid waste. Changing production and consumption habits in LMICs are expected to lead to increasing demand for agricultural and complex manufactured goods with a consequent increase in per capita waste generation in these countries (Scheinberg et al. 2010).

Waste management

In Europe waste management legislation and strategies are based on the fundamental concept of the waste hierarchy (see Table 8.2) in which the

Table 8.2 The waste hierarchy

Waste strategy	Description
Prevention (reduce)	Using less material in design and manufacture, keeping products for longer, re-use, using less hazardous materials.
Preparing for re-use	Checking, cleaning, repairing, refurbishing, whole items or spare parts.
Recycling	Turning waste into a new substance or product; includes composting if it meets quality protocols.
Other recovery	Includes anaerobic digestion,[1] incineration with energy recovery, gasification and pyrolysis which produce energy (fuels, heat and power) and materials from waste.
Disposal	Landfill and incineration without energy recovery.

[1] Anaerobic digestion is a treatment process which harnesses natural bacteria to produce biogas and a residue known as digestate, from waste biodegradable materials, such as agricultural manure and slurry, food waste and sewage sludge.

Source: After EU Waste Framework Directive (2008)

three 'Rs' of reduce, re-use and recycle are seen as a primary goal of any integrated, sustainable waste management system (Wilson et al. 2013). In the UK, for example, the waste hierarchy is explicit in legislation as well as in planning and environmental permitting regulations.

Waste prevention/minimization (reduce)

The ideal waste management strategy is not to produce any waste at all (Rodenbeck et al. 2010), thus prevention or minimization is seen as the highest aim of any waste management strategy (DEFRA 2007). The advantages of waste minimization include financial savings (reduced raw materials, water, energy, labour, handling, transport, waste treatment and waste disposal costs; improved operating efficiency and lower production costs); environmental benefits (more efficient use of materials, energy and water; reduced pollution to land, air and water; easier compliance with regulations); and company benefits (improved market position and public image and greater staff motivation).

Re-use

Products can be designed to be used a number of times before becoming obsolete. For example, food and drink containers or car tyres can be designed to be re-usable. Products can be re-used (or repaired) by another consumer and they can also be specifically designed to make re-use or recycling simpler through choice of components or method of construction or manufacture.

Re-use has advantages of savings in the energy and raw materials required to make new products, reduced waste disposal needs (and hence costs) and cost savings for consumers. Re-use may also create new market opportunities, for example, refillable products (such as dry foods, laundry liquid and other cleaning products).

Recycling

According to the principles of the waste hierarchy, at the end of a product's life, as many of the component materials as possible should be recovered. Several 'waste streams' have been earmarked for special concern. These include packaging waste, end-of-life vehicles, batteries and electrical and electronic waste. In Europe, Member States are required to introduce legislation on waste collection, re-use, recycling and disposal of these waste streams and several European Union countries already recycle over 50 per cent of packaging.

Recycling has a number of positive impacts:

- Reduce energy consumption (e.g. recycling aluminium saves 90 per cent of the energy associated with mining and extraction of aluminium ore as well as preventing CO_2 and SO_2 emissions and the production of bauxite waste).
- Preserve natural resources. For example, 1 million mobile phones if recycled can recover 35,274 pounds of copper, 772 pounds of silver, 75 pounds of gold and 33 pounds of palladium (EPA 2012).
- Create jobs and increase economic activity. For example, in many countries (particularly low-income countries) there are active informal and micro-enterprise based recycling, re-use and repair systems driven by the market value of the waste material and products (Wilson et al. 2013).

Key factors that hinder recycling include both individual and structural difficulties. For the individual the cost to the consumer at the market-place does not take account of the costs to the environment or health of managing the product when it becomes waste, nor are there currently many incentives for the consumer to separate used goods for recycling such as ease of recycling (e.g. doorstep collections), deposits paid back when goods are returned or charges levied for collection of waste that has not been recycled.

Other recovery

Biological waste treatment methods

Biowaste is the organic and biodegradable fraction of the waste stream including food waste, sewage sludge, manures and slurries. Biowastes can be treated via anaerobic digestion or though composting (when heat generated can be recovered) and they have the potential to be a source of renewable energy. Additionally, many carbon-rich composts and digestates that are derived from the treatment of biowastes can be used in agriculture to improve soil structure and as inorganic fertilizers.

In Europe, Directive 1999/31/EC on the landfill of waste has not only required a reduction in the total amount of waste going to landfill but also specifies a reduction in the amount of biodegradable municipal waste going to landfill (to 35 per cent by 2016). The introduction of landfill taxes in response to this legislation has been the primary driver towards increasing the recovery of organic material from waste, rising from 28 kg/capita in 1999 to 89 kg/capita in 2009 (Hartmut Schrör 2011).

Energy from waste (incineration)

Incineration (burning waste at high temperatures) reduces the volume of waste by up to 90 per cent and mass by up to 70 per cent, and generates heat and power. If done in a controlled manner, it destroys the organic contaminants and concentrates and immobilizes the inorganic contaminants (some of which may be recovered from bottom ash or slag). Modern incinerators are subject to stringent regulation and use advanced technology to reduce the emission of potentially hazardous byproducts of incomplete combustion such as dioxins and polycyclic aromatic hydrocarbons (Rodenbeck et al. 2010). However, uncontrolled incineration also occurs, and such 'backyard' burning can be a significant source of air pollution. As a result of the perceived toxicity of the byproducts of incineration, this option is often the subject of considerable public concern about health effects. In high-income countries, controlled incineration has increasingly become a key part of integrated sustainable waste management strategies (Scheinberg et al. 2010).

Disposal

Landfill

The aim of landfill as a waste disposal method is to use the natural processes of decomposition over long time periods to convert waste into harmless substances. The key requirement is to maintain the integrity of the landfill site while this process occurs so that any harmful byproducts of this decomposition process remain inside the site and do not migrate out to the wider environment.

In high-income countries, landfill is subject to strict technical standards and licensing in order to minimize environmental effects as well as to financial disincentives (such as landfill tax). While landfill is now seen as the last resort for biodegradable waste there remain some wastes for which landfill remains the best or most appropriate option, including:

- some hazardous wastes such as asbestos;
- low level and very low level radioactive waste;

- some 'inert' materials and wastes;
- to restore quarries and mineral workings;
- certain process residues, such as pre-treated industrial wastes from which no further resources can be recovered;
- waste for which the alternatives to landfill are not justified by economic cost, or environmental and resource efficiency benefits.

Many LMICs continue to dispose of their waste in open dumps or poorly operated landfills. Lower-income countries may struggle with the capital investment and technical capability required for more technologically advanced waste management.

Health effects of waste disposal

All waste management practices impact on health and the environment to a greater or lesser degree (see Box 8.1, based on Rodenbeck et al. 2010). Impacts may vary from direct exposure to chemical contamination from a dump or poorly controlled landfill site to indirect effects such as those mediated through global warming (to which waste management practices contribute, e.g. by methane produced by decomposing waste and by use of fossil fuels for transporting waste). Health effects may result from the specific composition of the waste itself (e.g. hazardous wastes with particular known health risks) or from issues common to all types of waste management such as road usage, fossil fuel consumption and nuisance issues such as noise, odour and litter. Clearly the potential health effects of waste are broad and complex and go beyond local effects of a specific waste site.

Box 8.1:   Health risks from waste

- Infectious disease risks from poorly managed solid waste.
- Contamination of drinking water and soil by biological, chemical and mining waste.
- Gas migration and leachate discharges from landfill.
- Emissions of air pollutants from incinerators.
- Contamination of food from waste chemicals that escape into the environment.

Studies on the health effects of waste disposal are specific to each disposal or management method used, as each method of waste management is likely to give rise to different pollutants and different exposure routes. The difficulties in assessing the health effects of waste disposal not only arise from methodological issues (such as measuring exposure and health outcomes; study design; control of confounding factors; and statistical power) but also from the paucity of epidemiological studies. Toxicological data may be available for specific contaminants but provide limited information on the likely human health impact of a complex environmental pollution source such as a waste site.

 Activity 8.2

In terms of exposure to waste, what are the main routes by which humans are exposed to contaminants from waste? Are there particular individuals who might be at greater risk to exposure from waste contaminants?

Feedback

In order for an individual to be exposed to waste products there must first be a source of contaminants (e.g. a smoke stack or a landfill site). The contaminant must have a means of travel between the source and the individual (or receptor), for example through dispersal into the air, or leaching into groundwater and soil. Such dispersed pollutants, however, can only harm health if there is a point of contact between the contaminant and the individual and the contaminant is able to enter the body (e.g. through inhalation, skin absorption or absorption through the digestive tract).

There are two kinds of populations who are more at risk from waste contaminants: those who have greater chance of exposure and those who are inherently more vulnerable to ill effects. Those who are more likely to be exposed are primarily those who work in waste disposal occupations whether formally or informally. Additionally communities living close to waste sites are more at risk of exposure than those who are further away (although probably at much lower levels than workers). Exposure to hazardous and complex wastes (such as electronic waste) may be a considerable distance from the point of origin of the waste and may even be in a different country.

Certain groups of individuals may be more susceptible to health effects of pollution and these include the elderly, the very young, pregnant women (and their unborn children) and those with pre-existing health conditions.

Incineration

The incineration process can result in three potential sources of exposure: (1) emissions to the atmosphere; (2) via solid ash residues; and (3) via cooling water. The byproducts of the combustion process may contain hazardous or toxic pollutants and emissions will add to background pollution levels. As a result, there is often considerable public concern over the possible health effects of living near to incinerators processing hazardous, clinical or municipal waste (DEFRA 2004). Provided that solid ash residues and cooling water are handled and disposed of appropriately it is likely that atmospheric emissions remain the only significant route of exposure to people (Maynard et al. 2010).

Incineration – evidence for health effects

Based on the individual pollutants known to arise from incinerator processes, it is possible to suggest the health effects which might be of concern. These include:

- cancers and birth defects due to exposure to dioxins, furans and polycyclic aromatic hydrocarbons;
- acute toxicity, cancer and reproductive effects due to heavy metal exposure;
- respiratory disease due to particulate exposure.

There have been few epidemiological studies that examine the health of communities living in close proximity to incinerators with the majority of published studies relating to the older generation of incinerators, which have been phased out through the introduction of stricter emission controls (DEFRA 2004). This is due to the long latency for some health outcomes studied (e.g. cancer) and hence is unavoidable, but does complicate the interpretation of such studies. Exposure to pollutants from uncontrolled burning of waste in LMICs is likely to be considerably higher than even older incinerators but there are few studies available which evaluate such health effects.

Further limitations of the epidemiology include:

- studies are often observational or ecological so cannot demonstrate a causal relationship;
- studies are primarily retrospective, often prompted by complaints about health 'clusters' and may therefore be open to bias;
- population sizes are often too small to detect statistically significant effects unless these are very large;
- inadequate control of confounding factors such as socioeconomic variables;
- exposure to other emissions, population variables and spatial/temporal issues;
- studies suffer from poor exposure assessment, often using distance as a proxy and not taking into account the influence of meteorology or technical processes.

A review of the health effects of waste management (DEFRA 2004) concluded:

> the published epidemiological studies of the health of communities living in the vicinity of incinerators have failed to establish a convincing link between incinerator emissions and adverse effects on public health; specifically no impact was demonstrated on the incidence of cancer, respiratory health symptoms or reproductive outcomes.

The UK Health Protection Agency review of health effects of air emissions from incinerators considered evidence on health effects of dioxins, polycyclic aromatic hydrocarbons, particulates and heavy metals and concluded that:

> modern, well managed incinerators make only a small contribution to local concentrations of air pollutants. It is possible that such small additions could have an impact on health but such effects, if they exist, are likely to be very small and not detectable.
>
> (Maynard et al. 2010)

However, those working in incinerators may be at risk of health effects from occupational exposure to products of combustion (Committee on Health Effects of Waste Incineration 2000).

Landfill

The key factor for human health when related to landfill is not what goes *into* the site, but what comes *out*. Preventing health effects relies on ensuring that what is inside the landfill remains inside. Figure 8.2 shows the possible routes of exposure to humans of material escaping from a landfill site. Additional health effects from operational processes such as transport of wastes, site security, worker health and safety and pests and vermin must all be considered. In low-income countries waste pickers on open dumps are subject to specific health hazards such as accidental injury and direct exposure to bacteria and air pollutants (Scheinberg et al. 2010).

Landfill – evidence for health effects

A key problem with assessing health effects from landfill sites is exposure assessment: characterizing who is exposed, to what substance and at what dose. The main issues are as follows.

- *What is the composition of the waste in the landfill?* In high-income countries and modern landfill sites this will be well documented but the subsequent changes in both physical and chemical composition as a result of decomposition processes are not well understood. In older and poorly regulated landfills or unregulated dumps this will be even less certain.

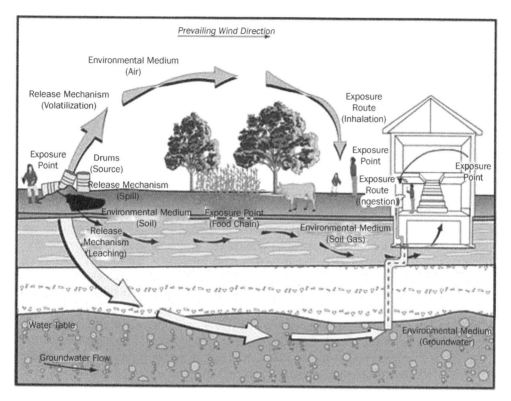

Figure 8.2 Exposure routes from landfill waste to humans.
Source: http://www.atsdr.cdc.gov/hac/PHAManual/ch6.html

- *What is the exposure route?* The type of chemical(s) which are escaping from the site, their method of transport through the environment and their likely end point is determined by the chemistry and physical form of the waste products in question and by local hydrogeology and climatic conditions.
- *What is the likely dose?* This is a factor not only of the chemical composition and physical form of the waste products escaping from a site but also of the characteristics of the local population such as proximity, density and land use.

Epidemiological studies have identified health outcomes associated with living near landfill sites, including congenital anomalies, low birth weight, cancer and non-specific health effects such as fatigue and headache (see e.g. Vrijheid 2000). A key difficulty with most studies is the lack of exposure data so that the proxy used for exposure is a simple 'distance from site' measure. Many of the studies are ecological and unable to take account of individual risk factors such as socioeconomic status or lifestyle factors. Risk estimates are typically small and it is difficult to separate effects due to confounding and bias and those which might be causally related to the hazard under consideration (HPA 2011).

After extensive review of the evidence, the UK Committee on Toxicity of Chemicals in Food, Consumer Products and the Environment concluded that further case control or cohort studies were required to investigate health effects around landfill sites (COT 2010). Both COT and the UK HPA (2011) consider that there is currently insufficient evidence to suggest that well managed landfill sites pose a risk to human health.

Health effects of other waste disposal practices

Other than landfill and incineration there have been few studies of the health effects of other waste management options. This may be partly because they do not appear to generate a great deal of public concern.

Materials recycling facilities may present a hazard due to biological materials, and particularly bioaerosols. The associated risks are similar to those occurring in a composting plant. There is evidence that compost derived from the organic fraction of municipal solid waste can contain metals and persistent organic pollutants, as well as microbial and fungi toxins (such as *Aspergillus*). There are also significant chemical and physical hazards to the worker in the recycling plant (which may extend beyond the boundaries of the plant), including exposure to vapours and suspended particulate matter.

A small number of studies of workers at recycling and composting plants have indicated an association with a variety of skin, respiratory and gastro-intestinal symptoms (DEFRA 2004), although not all studies show a positive association. A more recent review of health effects of composting sites noted that the available information around occupational risks, and/or the factors that produce those risks, was scarce (Domingo and Nadal 2009). Control of hazards associated with composting involves planning controls to limit the distance between the site and any sensitive receptors, and limiting the quantity of waste handled at any one time. There is little available evidence for specific health effects of other waste management practices other than occupational risks.

Global issues of waste management

Climate change

All waste management options have some impact on climate change. Landfill produces methane gas (CH_4) which is a greenhouse gas. Incineration leads to the production of another greenhouse gas, carbon dioxide (CO_2). Recycling can also contribute to climate change as it uses energy (fossil fuels) in the industrial processes. Composting also emits carbon dioxide and methane. However, waste disposal is a relatively minor contributor to global greenhouse gas (only 3–5 per cent of anthropogenic emissions). Additionally, waste management practices have the potential to reduce greenhouse gas emissions.

It should be noted that the issue of transport of goods for recycling, re-use and composting must be taken into account in the evaluation of the positive impact of these practices.

Environmental justice and waste

There is evidence that exposure to the negative impacts of waste varies by socioeconomic status in many countries. Waste facilities are often dispro-portionately located in areas with more deprived residents (Martuzzi et al. 2010). This applies to waste incinerators, landfills, hazardous waste sites and both legal and illegal disposal sites.

In addition, in LMICs unmanaged or poorly managed waste tends to have the greatest impact on the health of the poorest and most vulnerable. In some areas micro-economies develop that are based on the picking up of waste (whether collected or not) and selling on any reusable or recyclable material. Although such informal practices may be a vital part of waste management in developing countries, the health impacts for these workers include injury, intoxication and infection, and are often borne by the most vulnerable (primarily children) (Scheinberg et al. 2010). More recently the growing problem of electronic waste has led to the development of informal recycling centres in Asia and Africa where goods are collected, manually dismantled and openly burnt in order to recover metals. Workers (again primarily the most vulnerable: women, children and the elderly) are exposed to toxic fumes (e.g. polycyclic aromatic hydrocarbons, polyhydrochlorinated biphenyls and polybrominated diphenyl ethers) as well as heavy metals (such as mercury, lead and zinc) and injury (Noel-Brune et al. 2013).

The practice of exporting hazardous waste (also known as 'waste trafficking') for disposal in developing countries further exacerbates the existing problems faced by LMICs in managing their own waste. The dumping of hazardous wastes endangers individuals living or working near the sites as well as those further away (via contamination of the wider environment). If recycling and recovery is poorly managed it is less efficient, with consequent loss of natural resources. Additionally, such illegal and unsound treatment, by being cheaper, skews the market and hinders the development of safe and efficient waste management systems (Appeleqvist 2011).

Recognition of the transfer of waste as an issue of environmental justice led to the creation in 1989 of the Basel Convention on the Control of Trans-boundary Movements of Hazardous Wastes and Their Disposal. This was hailed as one of the most important steps taken in recent times towards the international regulation of hazardous waste. However, it allows legal transfer of waste between countries if the exporting state does not have the facilities, capacity or disposal sites in order to dispose of the waste; if the wastes are required as raw materials for recycling or recovery industries; and if the transfer of waste is in accordance with other criteria as designated by the countries involved. Thus, despite legal restrictions, the burden of waste management is still being shifted from the formal manufacturing sector in high-income countries to the informal sector in LMICs. Electronic wastes are a prime example: instead of investing in research and development to devise proper waste treatment and recycling methods which are environmentally benign, technologically advanced countries currently exploit loopholes in the regulations (e.g. the legally allowed trade in 'products for re-use without prior refurbishment'), thus relocating the burden of waste management through the global toxic waste trade.

Activity 8.3

Read the extract by Selvam (1994) and then give a summary of how Panaji hoped to achieve an efficient and sustainable waste management system.

An example of an integrated waste management system in a developing country

Panaji, the capital of Goa, is a small but well-developed town with a population of 42,915. Panaji Municipal Council (PMC) is responsible for the collection, transportation and disposal of solid wastes generated within the municipal limits. Households and establishments including hospitals, private nursing homes, restaurants, etc., deposit their wastes in communal waste storage bins, for subsequent collection (manual) and transportation to an undeveloped and unsanitary dumping site. A large number of waste pickers make their livelihood by collecting a variety of recyclable wastes from bins and the disposal site. Households (40 per cent) and restaurants (27 per cent) are the two major waste generators. About 1.8 tons, 8 per cent of total wastes, are collected daily by waste pickers for recycling.

The major issues raised by the community are: inadequate number and faulty design of bins, irregular clearing by PMC workers, and the wet and unhygienic conditions around the bins. Meetings with representatives of other major waste generators, restaurants, hospitals and nursing homes revealed their preference for a personalized 'door-to-door' system for restaurants and their willingness to pay for the improved service level.

The social survey findings formed an important basis for the development of a sustainable solid waste management model. For example, the Panaji survey provided some unexpected results; people in Panaji are not interested in 'door-to-door' collection of wastes; people are willing to make a monthly payment of Rs.10/- (US$ 1 = INR 31.80 6/94 rate) per *household for a communal primary waste collection system with an improved bin design and daily clearance through a mechanized system.*

Various disposal options such as composting, pelletization, incineration, etc. were evaluated. The potential for resource recovery and revenue generation influenced the decision for composting organic wastes from vegetable markets and restaurants.

Recommendations to improve the existing solid waste management situation:

- *Replace the existing bottomless cement concrete bins with suitable numbers of metallic bins, a minimum of one bin within 50 m of all households.*
- *Collect the restaurant wastes from 'door-to-door', twice a day, on a full cost recovery basis. The six existing closed body vehicles should be used for servicing 200 restaurants per day.*
- *Collect the infectious wastes separately from hospitals and nursing homes for incineration at the Goa Government Medical College Hospital, on a full cost recovery basis.*
- *Use the existing garbage compactor exclusively for collecting the organic wastes from the municipal market.*

Waste disposal:

- *Install a manual composting plant for processing eight tons of restaurant and market wastes every day. With proper marketing, it is not only possible to fully recover the production cost of Rs. 325/- per ton, but also possible to make a modest profit.*
- *Develop the abandoned laterite stone quarry pit into a sanitary landfill site. Improve the existing dump site operation (until the new site is developed) by spreading the waste and covering it with construction wastes using a hired bulldozer on a regular basis.*
- *Sustain the waste pickers' contribution to resource recovery, by organizing them into a formal group with the help of a local NGO, providing them with tools to sort out wastes, raising their status to that of waste collectors, and providing either free or low-cost medical facilities through the state health department.*

Feedback

In order to be sustainable, an integrated waste management scheme has to include all aspects of waste, from production to disposal. This strategy did not cover waste prevention, but did propose a cost-effective method of dealing with waste after consultation with businesses and communities. Consumers are prepared to pay to have a more efficient and hygienic service. Composting will make a profit and waste pickers will have improved livelihoods. The local authority was able to ensure that resources were used effectively and that the system maximized waste collection and its subsequent recycling or disposal.

Summary

Waste is produced as the result of domestic and industrial activity. There are a number of ways to deal with waste, including reduction, re-use, recycling, energy recovery and disposal. The waste hierarchy can help to establish the best and most environmentally efficient method for dealing with waste, leaving disposal as the least preferred option. Disposal methods have the potential to harm both the environment and human health if not properly designed or maintained. The study of waste on human health is complicated by the difficulties of establishing exposure routes and the often unknown nature of the contaminants. There remain inequities in impacts of waste disposal between countries.

References

Appelqvist, B. (2011) *International Solid Waste Association Position Paper on Waste Trafficking*. Vienna: ISWA.

Beck, E.C. (1979) The Love Canal tragedy, *United States Environmental Protection Agency Journal*, January, http://www2.epa.gov/aboutepa/love-canal-tragedy, accessed 25 October 2013.

Committee on Health Effects of Waste Incineration (2000) *Waste Incineration and Public Health*. Washington, DC: National Academy Press.

COT (Committee on Toxicity of Chemicals in Food, Consumer Products and the Environment) (2010) Second statement on landfill sites, http://cot.food.gov.uk/cotstatements/cotstatementsyrs/cotstatements2010/cot201001.

Contreras, F., Ishii, S., Aramaki, T., Hanaki, K. and Connors, S. (2010) Drivers in current and future municipal solid waste management systems: cases in Yokohama and Boston, e-pub 26 November 2009, *Waste Management Research*, January, 28(1): 76–93.

DEFRA (Department for Environment, Food and Rural Affairs) (2004) *Review of Environmental and Health Effects of Waste Management: Municipal Solid Waste and Similar Wastes.* Enviros Consulting Ltd and University of Birmingham with Risk and Policy Analysts Ltd, Open University and Maggie Thurgood. London: HMSO, https://www.gov.uk/government/uploads/system/uploads/attachment_data/file/69391/pb9052a-health-report-040325.pdf.

DEFRA (Department for Environment, Food and Rural Affairs) (2007) *Waste Strategy for England 2007*, http://archive.defra.gov.uk/environment/waste/strategy/strategy07/documents/waste07-strategy.pdf.

Domingo, J.L. and Nadal, M. (2009) Domestic waste composting facilities: a review of human health risks, *Environment International*, 35: 382–9.

EPA (2012) The secret life of a smartphone, https://www.epa.gov/sites/production/files/2015-06/documents/smart_phone_infographic_v4.pdf, accessed December 2013.

EU Framework Directive (2008) Directive 2008/98/EC of the European Parliament and of the Council of 19 November 2008 on waste and repealing certain directives, *Official Journal of the European Union*, 22 November, http://eur-lex.europa.eu/LexUriServ/LexUriServ.do?uri=OJ:L:2008:312:0003: 0030:en:PDF.

Hartmut Schrör (2011) Generation and treatment of waste in Europe 2008: Eurostat Statistics in focus 44/2011, EU 2011, http://epp.eurostat.ec.europa.eu/cache/ITY_OFFPUB/KS-SF-11-044/ EN/KS-SF-11-044-EN.PDF, accessed December 2013.

Hoornweg, D. and Bhada-Tata, P. (2012) *What a Waste: a global review of solid waste management*, Urban Development Series no. 15, World Bank, http://go.worldbank.org/BCQEP0TMO0.

HPA (2011) Impact on health of emissions from landfill sites RCE 18 July 2011, http://www.hpa.org. uk/webc/HPAwebFile/HPAweb_C/1309969974126.

Martuzzi, M., Mitis, F. and Forastiere, F. (2010) Inequalities, inequities, environmental justice in waste management and health, *European Journal of Public Health*, http://dx.doi.org/10.1093/eurpub/ ckp216.

Maynard, R.L., Walton, H., Pollitt, F. and Fielder, R. (2010) *The Impact on Health of Emissions to Air from Municipal Waste Incinerators*. London: HPA, http://www.hpa.org.uk/webc/HPAwebFile/HPAweb_ C/1251473372218.

Noel-Brune, M. et al. (2013) Health effects of exposure to e-waste, *Lancet Global Health*, 1(2): e70.

Rodenbeck, S., Orloff, K. and Falk, H. (2010) Solid and hazardous waste, in H. Frumkin (ed.) *Environmental Health: from global to local*, 2nd edn. San Francisco: Jossey-Bass.

Scheinberg, A., Wilson, D.C. and Rodic, L. (eds) (2010) *Solid Waste Management in the World's Cities*. London: Earthscan for UN HABITAT.

Selvam, P. (1994) Community-based SWM project preparation, 20th WEDC Conference, Colombo, Sri Lanka.

UNEP (2010) *Waste and Climate Change: global trends and strategy framework*. Nairobi: United Nations Environment Programme.

Vrijheid, M. (2000) Health effects of residence near hazardous waste landfill sites: a review of epidemiologic literature, *Environmental Health Perspective*, 108 (suppl. 1): 101–12.

Wilson, C. (2007) Development drivers for waste management, *Waste Management Research*, 25: 198–207.

Wilson, D.C., Velis, C.A. and Rodic, L. (2013) Integrated sustainable waste management in developing countries, *Proceedings of the ICE – Waste and Resource Management*, 166(2): 52–68.

Zaman, A.U. (2013) Identification of waste management development drivers and potential emerging waste treatment technologies, *International Journal of Environmental Science and Technology*, 10(3): 455–64.

The urban environment and health

Emma Hutchinson and James Milner

Overview

There are many environmental health issues associated with urban areas and urbanization (urban growth). This chapter considers the various health benefits and challenges of urbanization, and how these affect different populations within cities. The chapter then introduces the different aspects that comprise the urban environment and briefly considers the potential implications for health of each, with a particular focus on the physical environment. The chapter then evaluates the requirements necessary to create healthy cities, including those aspects of urban planning which promote sustainability. Lastly, a range of policy actions, including how cities might be designed for the optimal health of their inhabitants, are presented.

Learning objectives

By the end of this chapter you will be able to:

- appreciate the health issues associated with increasing urbanization
- discuss the health issues associated with urban environments
- compare the differential impact of urban environmental problems on the health of different groups within cities
- critically appraise the requirements for a healthy city

Key terms

Green spaces: Areas of grass, trees, or other vegetation set apart for recreational or aesthetic purposes or for the control of hazards (e.g. natural flood management) in an otherwise urban environment.

Infrastructure: The basic facilities, services and installations needed for the functioning of a community, such as transport and communication systems, water and power lines, schools, post offices and prisons.

Slum/informal settlement: Defined by the UN as informal housing that lacks at least one of the basic conditions of decent housing: adequate sanitation, improved water supply, durable housing or adequate living space.

Spatial planning: A more rational organization of land uses, and the linkages between them, than can be delivered by urban planning alone, balancing the demands for development with the need to protect the environment and to achieve social objectives (Economic Commission for Europe 2008).

Urban advantage: Potential benefits that urbanization brings for poverty reduction and/or health improvement (and its converse, urban disadvantage).

Urban area: Geographic area often defined as having a population of 10,000–50,000 or more.

Urban environment: The natural, built and institutional elements that determine the physical, mental and social health and wellbeing of people who live in cities and towns (ICSU 2011).

Urban penalty: Unequal access to economic resources that results in differing opportunities for health.

Urban planning: The body of knowledge on land use and design of the urban environment (including transportation networks) which aims to ensure the orderly development of urban communities.

Urban transition: Increasing proportion of a nation's population living in urban areas.

Urbanization: The increasing concentration of people and economic activities in towns and cities.

Obesogenic environment: The role environmental factors may play in determining both nutrition and physical activity leading to increased obesity (UK Government's Foresight Programme 2007).

Healthy cities: A healthy community in which all systems work well (and work together), and in which all citizens enjoy a good quality of life.

Introduction

In 1800, only 3 per cent of the world's population lived in urban areas. By 1900, this had risen to 14 per cent, although only 12 cities had 1 million or more inhabitants. In 2008, for the first time, the world's population was evenly split between urban and rural areas. There were more than 400 cities with over 1 million inhabitants and 19 with over 10 million. It is expected that 70 per cent of the world population will be urban by 2050, and that most urban growth will occur in low- and middle-income countries (LMICs).

Urban areas bring economies of scale and proximity to infrastructure, such as water provision and sanitation. Such services reduce the risks of injury, illness and premature death, which in addition to the improved education provision, employment opportunities and access to health care that exist in many urban areas, can be considered beneficial for health. However, in LMICs large sectors of society live in informal settlements, where conditions can be extremely poor and health burdens consequently very high, and these benefits tend to be spread much more unevenly than in cities in high-income countries.

The main driving force for urbanization is economic growth, particularly where manufacturing and services are the growth areas (see Chapter 3). Economic, political and social change such as natural disasters and conflict may also contribute to migration from rural areas.

One of the potential consequences of population influx into cities is that it may occur at a faster rate than infrastructural development can cope with, particularly in low-income countries where social and economic conditions are often uncoordinated. This situation may lead to a lack of adequate services, such as water supply and sanitation, lack of good quality housing and a resultant increase in inequality – all contributing to disadvantages to health if growth is poorly managed. Further discussion on policy responses to rapid urbanization is presented later in the chapter.

Although urbanization is covered in other chapters (5 and 7), urbanization increasingly affects so much of the world's population that it is useful to consider it in its own right. In the next sections, we will consider the different aspects of the urban environment, and how these relate to health.

The urban environment

The urban environment can be defined as 'the natural, built and institutional elements that determine the physical, mental and social health and wellbeing of people who live in cities and towns' (ICSU 2011). Cities are complex and dynamic systems whose physical, social and cultural environments, and socioeconomic aspects, interact and influence human health.

 Activity 9.1

This activity focuses on the physical, social and cultural, psychosocial and economic aspects of the urban environment. Complete Table 9.1 referring to any city with which you are familiar.

Table 9.1 Aspects of the urban environment

Aspect	Example (+ve)	Example (–ve)	Potential health effect	Prevention
Physical				
Social/cultural				
Psychosocial				
Economic				

1 Insert an example of one negative and one positive impact of each of the environmental influences.
2 Insert the likely health effect (for the negative example) in each case.
3 Suggest a possible method of prevention of the negative health effect.

Feedback

Table 9.2 shows some examples of the answers you might have included, though there are many others.

Table 9.2 Aspects of the urban environment (completed)

Aspect	Example (+ve)	Example (–ve)	Potential health effect	Prevention
Physical	Improved sanitation	Air pollution from transport	Respiratory and cardio-vascular disease	Reduce car numbers, provide better public transport
Social/cultural	Education	Lack of physical security (e.g. risk of break-ins)	Violence	Improve social cohesion
Psychosocial	Access to leisure facilities	Overcrowding	Mental health problems	Better-quality housing
Economic	Employment opportunities	High cost of housing	General health	Encourage industry and services to relocate

Physical aspects of the urban environment

Physical aspects of the urban environment that have an effect on population health include water supply and quality, sanitation provision, industrial and residential pollution, housing, infrastructure and the city's geographical situation (e.g. on a floodplain or an earthquake belt).

The infrastructure accompanying increased urbanization includes both an increase in roads and an increase in road transport. Road transport has two important physical influences: first, it is the major source of air pollution, and, second, motor vehicles cause accidental injuries (see Chapter 7). On the other hand, well-designed infrastructure may improve access to services, employment and health care. In many cities 30–60 per cent of the population lives in overcrowded, poor quality housing, with implications for the spread of airborne infections and exposure to heat, cold and damp (see Chapter 6). Indoor air pollution can cause acute respiratory infections in children and chronic lung disease in adults.

The largest growth in urbanization is in LMICs, many of which have tropical climates that exaggerate environmental changes. For example, rainfall is heavier than in non-tropical regions, causing greater problems with run-off and sedimentation. Many cities in LMICs are not in suitable sites for expansion, with swamps, rivers, steep slopes or otherwise unsuitable topography restricting their growth. For example, Kingston, Jamaica, is situated in an area subject to seismic disturbances and intense tropical storms; these can lead to additional environmental problems and potential disaster for the citizens (Gupta and Asher 1998).

Social, socioeconomic and cultural aspects of the urban environment

Living in urban centres can offer great potential gains, such as access to paid work, education and cultural, recreational and health care facilities (sometimes referred to as the 'urban advantage'). However, in many cities, particularly in LMICs, growth in some sectors of the urban population is synonymous with the growth of urban poverty. This is the result of unequal access to economic resources and differing opportunities for health according to an individual's standing in the community (with respect to their income or occupation), and leads to health inequalities (the 'urban penalty').

An increase in the urban population due to migration from rural areas and high birth rates can lead to rapid urban growth beyond the service capacity of urban governments. This creates a situation where poverty is reinforced by lack of basic housing, services and employment infrastructure. Urban migration also occurs between countries; economic migrants move from low-income to higher-income countries. Social inequalities are recognized to influence transport patterns (such as car ownership, use of public transport), access to green space, pollution effects, housing quality, community participation and social isolation (WHO 2008).

The impact on health of the urban environment

Table 9.3 illustrates some specific impacts of the urban environment on health and the multi-factorial environmental causes or exacerbating factors. These impacts on health may be direct or indirect, beneficial or disadvantageous.

Table 9.3 The urban environment and associated specific health effects

Diseases	Socioeconomic environment	Physical environment	Behavioural, lifestyle
Communicable – acute respiratory infections	Overcrowding – e.g. sharing accommodation to reduce rental costs	Air pollution; house site; ventilation; house dust; building materials; damp; heating materials	Tobacco smoking; cooking and heating practice; level of use of health services; occupation
Communicable – diarrhoeal diseases	Cost of water; education of mother; access to individual water supply	Water quality; water source; excreta disposal	Hygiene behaviour; weaning practice; use of health services; water storage
Non-communicable – accidents	Maternal care – (working) mothers not having time to look after children; crowding – constraints of space for cooking, lack of access to childcare facilities for poor families	Road – density of traffic; Home – repair of house; cooking site; cooking materials	Cooking practice, occupation; maternal care patterns; cultural practices
Non-communicable diseases e.g. diabetes, heart disease	Low income; level of education and awareness	Obesogenic environments; lack of green space; lack of opportunities for active travel	Reliance on mechanized transport; diet
Psychosocial – mental distress	Living in a shanty area; insecurity of tenure; migration status; insecurity of income; unemployment	Quality of housing; physical security of area; child recreation facilities	Lack of self-esteem (related to employment and life circumstances); migration status; cultural conflict; gender; socioeconomic frustration

Source: After Landon (2006)

The direct benefits to health of living in an urban environment include access to a clean water supply, sanitation and waste collection, along with indirect benefits arising from the provision of infrastructure and health care, access to education and employment opportunities, and transport and recreational services. However, the concentration of people and the increased demands on the sectors on which they rely can also lead to adverse health effects. These can arise from increased air pollution from household cooking and heating (see Chapter 6) and from transport and industry, increased exposure to road traffic injuries, and increased exposure to noise (Kjellstrom et al. 2007) (see Chapter 7). In addition, existing patterns of urban planning and transport are associated in all areas (but particularly in high-income countries) with sedentary lifestyles, diminished space and opportunities for physical activity, and a consequent increase in related non-communicable diseases such as diabetes and cardiovascular disease (UK Government Foresight Programme 2007; WHO/UNEP Health and Environment Linkages Initiative 2012). There is also emerging research on the role of obesogenic environments (NICE 2014), which we will touch on later in the chapter.

Additionally, where urban growth is poorly managed this can result in poor quality housing with lack of sanitation and inadequate water supply, which leads to increased spread of communicable disease. These effects are exacerbated where inequalities exist (such as in informal housing or in areas in poverty), and can include social problems such as lack of security and social cohesion, and decreased access to health care provision and fresh food. This is common in low-income countries, but also can occur in high-income countries.

The impact of the urban environment on physical activity

There is evidence to suggest that the shift to more sedentary leisure time activities and less active forms of transport that are associated with urban

Table 9.4 Health benefits of regular physical activity

- Reduces the risk of dying prematurely from cardiovascular diseases (e.g. coronary heart disease and stroke).
- Reduces the risk of developing non-insulin dependent diabetes.
- Reduces the risk of developing high blood pressure.
- Reduces hypertension in those already with hypertension.
- Reduces the risk of developing colon cancer.
- Reduces the risk of developing breast cancer.
- Reduces the development of osteoarthritis and osteoporosis.
- Reduces fall-related injuries among older adults.
- Helps maintain a healthy weight and reduces overweight and obesity.
- Helps build and maintain healthy bones, muscles and joints.
- Reduces feelings of depression and anxiety and promotes physiological and psychological wellbeing.

Source: Adapted from WHO (2009), BHF (2011)

environments has led to an increase in the prevalence of obesity and non-communicable diseases, particularly in people from socially and economically disadvantaged backgrounds (UK Government Foresight Programme 2007; Allender et al. 2011). This is the case in high-income countries, but also applies to varying degrees in emerging economies (notably Mexico). Regular physical activity has multiple health benefits which are described in Table 9.4.

Reduced all-cause and cardiovascular mortality has been observed in those who frequently cycle and/or use walking as a mode of active transport (Shephard 2008), and a recent systematic review on the health effects of active travel showed modest benefits for health outcomes including all-cause mortality and hypertension, and suggestive evidence for diabetes prevention (Saunders et al. 2013).

The impact of the urban environment on social and psychological health

Components of the urban environment can have both negative and positive impacts on social and psychological health. Negative impacts include those arising from antisocial behaviours such as crime. There can also be direct negative social impacts from poor urban planning, such as community severance due to road building or heavy road traffic. For example, in many US cities there have been direct social impacts when infrastructures like highways are constructed in locations that divide existing communities.

Positive impacts at the individual level have been associated with community support for mental health and positive states of physiological wellbeing. At the community level, in areas with more supportive social networks, positive impacts on social capital and social inclusion are indicated (WHO 2009). There are different definitions of social capital, but they all share the idea that social networks have value for their members, arising from the benefits derived from cooperation between individuals and groups. Shared interests can be used to create, maintain and develop social networks – for example, community gardening groups, or support groups which provide information such as cancer support. Research has shown that individuals who are embedded in a network or community rich in support, social trust, information and norms – i.e. those who have high social capital – also have resources that help achieve health goals (Lin 2001).

The benefits of healthy urban environments

Having considered the impacts that aspects of the urban environment can have on health, we now consider which of those aspects are important in facilitating healthy urban environments – i.e. those in which we would wish to live, work and play. Evidence shows that the urban environment has a profound influence on the wider determinants of health. Tackling public health problems such as obesity, heart disease, stroke and mental health, and tackling inequalities in health, all involve remedies that go beyond the health sector and rely on the provision of healthier urban environments, in addition to the role of the economy and other government departments.

In a review of evidence for the WHO, four components of the spatial determinants of health in urban areas were identified: land use pattern; transport; green space; and urban design (Grant et al. 2009). The nature of the built environment, and particularly urban planning, affects the determinants of health in urban settings. These determinants include the ability of people to make healthy choices, for example, through the ability to use active transport; to have access to healthy food; and to be part of a supportive community (WHO Collaborating Centre for Healthy Urban Environments 2012).

A shift from an urban disadvantage to an urban advantage, where health outcomes in cities have improved in comparison to rural areas, has been shown (Rydin et al. 2012). However, this concept of urban advantage has also been criticized for assuming that further economic growth and urbanization in low-income countries will replicate the positive health outcomes that this has generated in high-income countries. Additionally, this concept does not allow for the range of health outcomes within cities – where the burden of ill health is often unevenly distributed among different sectors of the population (Rydin et al. 2012). Although there is compelling evidence to suggest that urban areas experience 'better' health than rural areas, the urban advantage will not be maintained without good governance and appropriate management of the urban environment.

Attention has been directed to urban planning, to whether form and structure have an impact on health and, if so, how these occur. Critical questions have been asked such as: What are the impacts of ongoing car-dependent

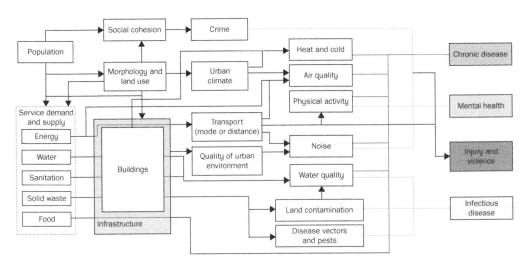

Figure 9.1 Health outcomes and the urban environment: connections.

Source: Rydin et al. (2012).

urbanization? What might be the impacts of higher dwelling densities? What relationships underlie these impacts? How can we identify causal factors and influences? How can planning be reformed to diminish adverse health impacts from urban systems? (Mead et al. 2006). The relationship between aspects of the urban environment and potential health outcomes are illustrated in Figure 9.1.

You can see that the relationship between physical factors such as energy, water and sanitation provision, urban planning (e.g. transport), quality of the urban environment (e.g. air quality, noise) and health outcomes is interrelated and complex. Research in these areas is ongoing.

Inequalities in urban areas

As described in the introduction to this chapter, the world's population is growing and more people are living in cities. The UN's Millennium Development Goal (MDG) 7 ('Ensure Environmental Sustainability') of improving the lives of at least 100 million slum dwellers has already been achieved (see Chapter 3). However, although the share of the urban population living in slums has declined, the absolute number of slum dwellers in low- and middle-income countries (LMICs) has grown.

Slums and squatter settlements represent a series of trade-offs between poor living quality and close proximity to jobs and markets, with no access to infrastructure and the informal and intermittent supply of urban services. The extract in Box 9.1 by Lanegran (1999) describes the rise in slum development in Mumbai, India, and the largely failed attempts to rectify the problem. Living on the margins does not necessarily mean a breakdown of social organization; squatter settlements can be stable communities with strong community organization and the provision of cheap or informal labour to support the national economy. The high population density in many poor urban areas means that small-scale interventions can assist many people and existing infrastructure can sometimes be upgraded to meet health demands (Kjellstrom et al. 2007).

Box 9.1:   Slums in Mumbai, India

The city of Mumbai is based on the island of Bombay in the west of India and has one of the world's best natural harbours. It is India's second largest, but most modern city. Slums (zopadpattis) have always existed in Mumbai. When the original fort was developed, the native villages moved close to the centre as squatter settlements. There was no planning, construction of infrastructure or implementation of facilities such as water, sewage, and drainage. Over the passage of time, this has led to problems for Mumbai's poor population. Mumbai has a very dense population with 16,500 people per square mile and a scarcity of housing. . .

... The scarcity of housing has meant the slums have spread wherever they can find space, including onto roads. Conditions are difficult. Inhabitants have to deal with issues such as constant migration, lack of water, no sewage or solid waste facilities, lack of public transport, pollution and housing shortages. Infant mortality in these areas is high as there are no amenities in rural India. General Hospitals in the Greater Mumbai region are overcrowded and under-resourced. There is either too little water in the area for drinking and sanitation, or in the monsoon season too much water and flooding.

There have been attempts by the government to improve the slum areas but they are difficult to implement successfully. For example, in 1985, the Slum Upgradation Project aimed to offer secure, long-term, legal plot tenure to slum households if they agreed to invest in their housing. The programme managed to target only the 10–12 per cent of the slum population who were capable of upgrading their homes. It offered no incentive for those without homes. Despite the attempts to remedy the slum problem of Mumbai, the slums are still growing.

(Lanegran 1999)

Since Lanegran wrote this piece, there have been attempts to address some of these problems, for example efforts to provide access to adequate sanitation (one toilet per 50 people). Toilet blocks are run by local community organizations, with fees to cover regular maintenance. However, evidence exists that not everyone is able to pay the fees, with the poorest among the population still having to resort to open defecation (based on McFarlane 2008, taken from Rydin et al. 2012).

However, the problem of sanitation and wastewater provision is not unique to low-income countries. In some cities in high-income countries, such as London, UK, problems can occur under certain conditions. The combined sewer network directs both sewage and rainwater to sewage treatment plants. At times of heavy rainfall, untreated raw sewage overflows directly into the River Thames and, with a growing population living and working in the city and a potentially increasing frequency of heavy rainfall with climate change, this issue may become a major public health and environmental concern (Rydin et al. 2012).

Activity 9.2

This activity about health inequalities within the urban environment in a low-income country is designed to help you to think about which sectors of society benefit from the urban advantage, which do not, and why.

Table 9.5 illustrates how the health of the population varies between and within urban and rural populations in Kenya. Describe and explain the differences in mortality rates between the groups. Think about vulnerable groups, particularly women and children, and consider what health issues arise for these groups in urban areas and why.

Table 9.5 Mortality and morbidity in children in urban and rural populations in Kenya

Location	Infant mortality (per 1,000)	Under 5 mortality rate (per 1,000)	Prevalence of diarrhoea with blood in children under 3 in two weeks prior to interview (%)
Kenya (rural and urban)	74	112	3.0
Rural	76	113	3.1
Nairobi	39	62	3.4
Other urban	57	84	1.7
Informal settlements in			
Nairobi	91	151	11.3
Kibera	106	187	9.8
Embakasi	164	254	9.1

Source: APHRC (2002)

Feedback

Where urbanization has been well managed (adequate provision of good quality housing, infrastructure and services), there tends to be benefits to health and wealth. However, the converse is also true. Your answers should have covered some of the following aspects.

There is a large difference in health outcomes between formal and informal (slum) settlements. For example, in Nairobi the overall prevalence of diarrhoea in children is 3.4 per cent, compared to 11.3 per cent in informal settlements. In low-income countries, some groups (e.g. women and children, and those already sick) are more susceptible to infectious and parasitic diseases (particularly diarrhoeal diseases and acute respiratory infections) due to the proportion of time spent in inadequate housing lacking sanitation and adequate water for personal hygiene, and poor nutrition. Additionally these groups have greater exposure to black smoke from biomass burning for cooking purposes (see Chapter 6).

The poor are more severely affected than the rich in terms of health outcomes, however the disparity in health outcomes between rich and poor not only occurs in low-income cities or cities in transition; the same gradient (although less steep) is found in high-income cities such as London.

In addition to lack of access to basic amenities and adequate living space, access to education, employment, a good diet and occupational safety are also important, and are frequently inequitably available to the urban poor.

Policy actions to promote healthy cities

Planning for healthy cities can help to manage environmental transitions so as to effect the most beneficial outcome for the environment and for health. Table 9.6 illustrates how urban environmental issues are dealt with in cities with different levels of income, and how cities with high incomes have the potential to establish healthy environments.

Policy solutions to achieve healthy cities in high-income countries

The impact of the urban or built environment on physical and mental health is seen through issues such as obesity, climate change, access to good quality local food, community infrastructure, air quality and noise pollution. For example, the UK government reports *Tackling Obesities* (2007) and *Healthy Weight, Healthy Lives* (2008) made clear links between obesity and the built environment. There is evidence that policies which increase active travel (e.g. walking and cycling) can have a large beneficial impact on a range of health outcomes, including reductions in obesity, diabetes and chronic heart and lung disease (Shepherd 2008; Woodcock 2009; ICSU 2011). However, in many cities, failure to consider this has resulted in an urban environment that makes it difficult for people to move easily around the city. There is sometimes tension between the development of mass transport systems and the ownership of private vehicles which leads to reduced investment in public transport, and therefore reduced active transport and potentially, may contribute to obesogenic environments (ICSU 2011).

Spatial planning (as introduced earlier in the chapter) intends to ensure better coordination between policies that can have an impact on community health. These include policies on employment and the economy, education, transport, health care provision, energy, waste, housing and the green and natural environment. These factors interact to influence urban health risks which, in addition to communicable and non-communicable disease, include physical activity levels, social impacts, air pollution, noise and unintentional injury (Grant et al. 2009).

Provision of green spaces

The provision of green space in urban areas is important to facilitate physical activity and can have health benefits for mental health and psychological

Table 9.6 Urban environmental issues and development

Sector or problem area	Low-income countries	Lower-middle-income countries	Upper-middle-income countries	High-income countries
Water supply service	Low coverage, high bacteria contamination, inadequate quantity for hygiene (high risk of food contamination and infectious diseases)	Low access by poor residents and informal neighbourhoods	Generally reliable, but rising demand causing shortages in resource supply	Good supply but high total consumption; some concern with trace pollutants
Sanitation	Very low coverage, open defecation in some neighbourhoods and low ratio public toilets to residents; high risk of diarrhoeal diseases	Better coverage of latrines and public toilets, but poorly maintained; low sewerage coverage	More access to improved sanitation, but still large numbers of residents in large cities not covered, especially in informal settlements; most wastewater discharge untreated	Full coverage; most wastewater treated
Solid waste management	Little organized collection; recycling by informal sector, open dumping or burning of mixed wastes; high exposure to disease vectors (rats, flies)	Moderate coverage of collection service, little separation of hazardous waste; mostly uncontrolled landfills	Better organized collection; severe problems but growing capacity for hazardous waste management; semi-controlled landfills	Increased emphasis on total waste reduction, resource recovery and preventing hazardous waste; controlled landfills or incineration
Air pollution	Indoor and ambient air pollution from low-quality fuels for household uses and power generation	Growing ambient air pollution from industrial and vehicular emissions (high per-vehicle, due to inefficient fuels and vehicles)	Ambient air pollution still serious (but greater capacity to control especially industrial sources)	Ambient air pollution mainly from vehicles (due to high volume of vehicle kilometres)

Table 9.6 Urban environmental issues and development (Continued)

Sector or problem area	Low-income countries	Lower-middle-income countries	Upper-middle-income countries	High-income countries
Land management (environmental zoning of fragile sites and preparation for new settlements)	Uncontrolled land development; intense pressure from squatter settlements on open sites	Ineffective or inappropriate land-use controls, pushing new settlements toward urban periphery; continued high population growth	Some environmental zoning	Regular use of environmental zoning; little population growth, but rising incomes press for more land consumption for existing residents
Accident risk	In-home and workplace accidents due to crowding, fires	Increased risks of industrial workplace and traffic accidents (pedestrians and non-motorized vehicles)	Transport accidents increasing, but some mitigation and emergency treatment response	Rate of industrial and transport accidents reduced despite increasing travel (vehicle kilometres)
Disaster management	Natural disasters produce massive loss of life and property especially in settlements in disaster-prone areas; little capacity for mitigation or emergency response	Somewhat better than in low-income, although with increasing risk of industrial disasters	Increasing awareness and capacity for disaster mitigation and emergency response	Good capacity for mitigation and response

Note: Cities grouped by estimated city product (city average income calculated by national accounts methods). Sample is of cities (including in OECD countries) with available data and is not statistically representative. Low income defined as city product below $750 per capita a year; lower-middle as $751–2,499; upper-middle as $2,500–9,999; high as above $10,000.

Source: World Bank (2003)

wellbeing (Allender et al. 2011). There is also some evidence to suggest that there are benefits for physical health in terms of reducing obesity (Lachowycz and Jones 2011). It is important that local authorities facilitate necessary maintenance and provide adequate security through environmental design of such features to minimize criminal activities, as if they are not adequately serviced they may turn into zones of fear avoided by many citizens (NICE 2006; WHO 2010). Other initiatives such as tree planting can have a number of benefits and there is wide scope for urban gardens, both private and communal, to provide fresh food for residents.

Planning for a healthy city – future directions

The WHO is committed to a long-term initiative aimed at improving the health and wellbeing of those who live and work in cities – the Healthy Cities Programme (WHO 1999). This states that if cities are to grow and prosper in a sustainable way, they will have to:

- reduce inequalities in health status and the determinants of health;
- develop public policies at the local level to create physical and social environments that support health;
- strengthen community action for health;
- help people develop new skills for health compatible with these approaches;
- reorient health services in accordance with policy.

These aspects have been further developed by the WHO Collaborating Centre for Healthy Urban Environments (2012) to include planning policy which considers such emerging issues as climate change, access to fresh food, safety and social cohesion, physical exercise, and local employment. These are mapped to the different aspects of the urban environment in Table 9.7.

The WHO initiative for healthy cities has shown the need for multi-sectoral cooperation for urban development projects. Attention needs to be paid to the quality of individual neighbourhoods as well as to service provisions within the city as a whole; the ability to buy adequate and safe food, to find a job, to gain education as well as access to health and other services are all as important as the availability of decent housing.

Since the inception of the WHO Healthy Cities Programme, a joint commission by the *Lancet* and University College London (UCL) has built on the Healthy Cities foundations to produce recommendations to policy-makers on how they can develop urban areas to foster the health of citizens so that they become healthy cities. These take into account the complex and unique nature of different cities and propose a new approach to the analysis and promotion of urban health, consisting of three components (*Lancet* 2012; Rydin et al. 2012):

- the promotion of experimentation to understand how to improve health in specific contexts;
- the application of strengthened assessments based on dialogue, deliberation and discussion between key stakeholders (rather than sole reliance on public health assessments);
- the creation of inclusive forums to debate the moral and ethical dimensions of different approaches to urban health.

Table 9.7 Healthy urban planning objectives

Aspects of the urban environment and determinants of health and wellbeing areas	Objectives for healthy urban planning
People	• Providing for the needs of all groups in the population • Reducing health inequalities • Health services for all
Lifestyle	• Promoting active travel • Promoting physically active recreation • Facilitating healthy food choices
Community	• Facilitating social networks and social cohesion • Supporting a sense of local pride and cultural identity • Promoting a safe environment
Economy	• Promoting accessible job opportunities for all sections of the population • Encouraging a resilient and buoyant local economy
Activities	• Reducing transport-related greenhouse gas emissions • Reducing building-related greenhouse gas emissions • Promoting substitution of renewable energy for fossil fuel use • Adapting of the environment to climate change
Built environment	• Ensuring good quality and supply of housing • Promoting a green urban environment supporting mental wellbeing • Planning an aesthetically stimulating environment, with acceptable noise levels • Road safety
Natural environment	• Promoting good air quality • Ensuring security and quality of water supply and sanitation • Ensuring soil conservation and quality • Reducing risk of environmental disaster
Global ecosystems	• Reducing transport-related greenhouse gas emissions • Reducing building-related greenhouse gas emissions • Promoting substitution of renewable energy for fossil fuel use • Adapting of the environment to climate change

Source: After Grant et al. (2009), WHO (2010)

Summary

The urban environment comprises the physical, social and economic dimensions. This chapter has explored the health effects that are associated with urban areas and differing health outcomes for city populations in high-, middle- and low-income countries. The potential problems associated with the process of urbanization have been considered, particularly in low-income countries, and some actions necessary to address these reviewed. Most cities, whether in high-income or low-income countries, exist with social and health inequalities between inhabitants. There can be an 'urban advantage' for health, but this is dependent on good governance. The chapter concluded by considering the WHO recommendations for planning healthy cities and evaluated the impacts on health of urban design and planning.

References

APHRC (2002) *Population and Health Dynamics in Nairobi's Informal Settlements*. Nairobi: African Population and Health Research Center.

Allender, S. et al. (2011) Policy change to create supportive environments for physical activity and healthy eating: which options are the most realistic for local government?, *Health Promotion International*, 18: 1–14.

BHF (British Heart Foundation) (2011) *Start Active, Stay Active: a report on physical activity for health from the four home countries*, http://www.bhfactive.org.uk/userfiles/Documents/startactivestay-active.pdf, accessed 28 September 2015.

Economic Commission for Europe (2008) *Spatial Planning: key instrument for development and effective governance with special reference to countries in transition*. Geneva: United Nations, http://www.unece.org/fileadmin/DAM/hlm/documents/Publications/spatial_planning.e.pdf, accessed 3 February 2013.

Lancet (2012) Editorial: Shaping cities for health: a UCL/*Lancet* Commission, *Lancet*, 30 May, doi:10.1016/S0140-6736(12)60870-8.

Grant, M., Barton, H., Coghill, N. and Bird, C. (2009) *Evidence Review on the Spatial Determinants of Health in Urban Settings*. Bonn: WHO European Centre for Environment and Health, http://www.architecturecentre.co.uk/assets/files/EvidenceBriefings/Spatial%20Determinants%20of%20Health%20in%20Urban%20Settings%20Briefing%20P1%20Overview.pdf, accessed 31 October 2012.

Gupta, A. and Asher, M. (1998) *Environment and the Developing World: principles, policies and management*. Chichester: John Wiley & Sons Ltd.

ICSU (2011) *Report of the ICSU Planning Group on Health and Wellbeing in the Changing Urban Environment: a systems analysis approach*. Paris: International Council for Science.

Kjellstrom, T., Friel, S., Dixon, J. et al. (2007) Urban environmental health hazards and health equity, *Journal of Urban Health: Bulletin of the New York Academy of Medicine*, 84(1): i86–97.

Lachowycz, K. and Jones, A.P. (2011) Obesity prevention, Greenspace and obesity: a systematic review of the evidence, *Obesity Reviews*, 12: e183–9.

Landon, M. (ed.) (2006) *Environmental Health and Sustainable Development*. Maidenhead: Open University Press.

Lanegran, D. (1999) Geography of world urbanisation course, http://www.macalester.edu/courses/geog61/espencer/slums.html.

Lin, N. (2001) Building a network theory of social capital, in N. Lin, K. Cook and R.S. Burt (eds) *Social Capital: theory and research*, pp. 3–29. New York: Aldine de Gruyter.

McFarlane, C. (2008) Sanitation in Mumbai's informal settlements: state, slum and infrastructure, *Environment and Planning*, 40: 88–107.

Mead, E., Dodson, J. and Ellway, C. (2006) *Urban Environments & Health: identifying key relationships & policy imperatives*, http://www.griffith.edu.au/__data/assets/pdf_file/0011/48647/urp-rm10-mead-et-al-2006.pdf, accessed 13 November 2012.

NICE (National Institute for Health and Care Excellence) (2006) *Physical Activity and the Environment: review two: urban planning and design*. London: NICE Public Health Collaborating Centre – Physical Activity, www.nice.org.uk/nicemedia/live/11679/34748/34748.doc, accessed 21 November 2012.

NICE (National Institute for Health and Care Excellence) (2014) *Obesity: identification, assessment and management of overweight and obesity in children, young people and adults*, https://www.nice.org.uk/guidance/cg189, accessed 28 September 2015.

Rydin, Y., Bleahu, A., Davies, M. et al. (2012). Shaping cities for health: complexity and the planning of urban environments in the 21st century, *Lancet*, 30 May, doi:10.1016/S0140-6736(12)60435-8.

Saunders, L.E., Green, J.M., Petticrew, M.P., Steinbach, R. and Roberts, H. (2013) What are the health benefits of active travel? A systematic review of trials and cohort studies, *PLoS ONE*, 8(8): e69912, doi:10.1371/journal.pone.0069912.

Shephard, R.J. (2008) Is active commuting the answer to population health?, *Sports Medicine*, 38(9): 751–8.

UK Government (2008) *Healthy Weight, Healthy Lives: a cross-government strategy for England*, http://webarchive.nationalarchives.gov.uk/20130401151715/http://www.education.gov.uk/publications/eOrderingDownload/DH-9087.pdf, accessed 28 September 2015.

UK Government Foresight Programme (2007) *Tackling Obesities: future choices – obesogenic environments – evidence review*, http://www.bis.gov.uk/assets/bispartners/foresight/docs/obesity/03.pdf, accessed 21 February 2011.

WHO (1999) Creating healthy cities in the 21st century, in D. Satterthwaite (ed.) *The Earthscan Reader on Sustainable Cities*, pp. 137–72. London: Earthscan Publications.

WHO (2008) *Closing the Gap in a Generation: health equity through action on the social determinants of health. Final report of the Commission on Social Determinants of Health*. Geneva: WHO.

WHO (2009) *Global Health Risks: mortality and burden of disease attributable to selected major risks*. Geneva: WHO.

WHO (2010) *Urban Planning, Environment and Health. From evidence to policy action, meeting report*. Denmark: WHO Regional Office for Europe, http://www.euro.who.int/__data/assets/pdf_file/0004/114448/E93987.pdf, accessed 21 November 2012.

WHO Collaborating Centre for Healthy Urban Environments (2012) Why is a healthy urban environment important?, http://www.bne.uwe.ac.uk/who/why.asp, accessed 31 October 2012.

WHO/UNEP Health and Environment Linkages Initiative (2012) The urban environment, http://www.who.int/heli/risks/urban/urbanenv/en/, accessed 13 November 2012.

Woodcock, J. (2009) Public health benefits of strategies to reduce greenhouse-gas emissions: urban land transport, *Lancet*, 374: 1930–43.

World Bank (2003) Urban environmental issues and development, in *World Development Report 2003: sustainable development in a dynamic world*. Washington, DC: World Bank.

Disasters 10

Virginia Murray and Sari Kovats

Overview

Disasters are a serious disruption of the functioning of a community involving widespread human, material, economic or environmental losses and impacts. Disasters, by definition, are events that exceed the ability of the affected community to cope using its own resources. Disasters may have natural or technological causes, and have serious implications for health (deaths, injuries, infectious diseases, chemical contamination and psychosocial effects). The health effects that occur will depend on the type of disaster, where the disaster took place and the population's capacity to cope. Public health strategies have been developed to reduce the health impacts of disasters, both before (preparedness), during and after (response) an event occurs.

Learning objectives

By the end of this chapter you will be able to:

- describe the types and causes of natural and technological disasters
- describe the health implications of natural and technological disasters
- understand the role of public health in disaster preparedness and response
- understand how environmental change may affect disaster risk in the future

Key terms

Disaster: Severe alterations in the normal functioning of a community or a society due to hazardous physical events interacting with vulnerable social conditions, leading to widespread adverse human, material, economic or environmental effects which require immediate emergency response to satisfy critical human needs and that may require external support for recovery.

Disaster preparedness: Activities and measures taken in advance to ensure effective response to the impact of hazards, including issuing timely and effective early warnings and the temporary evacuation of people and property from threatened locations.

Disaster risk management: Processes for designing, implementing and evaluating strategies, policies and measures to improve the understanding of disaster risk and promote disaster risk reduction. Also to promote continuous improvement in disaster preparedness, response and recovery practices, with the explicit purpose of increasing human security, wellbeing, quality of life and sustainable development.

Disaster risk reduction: Activities and measures that aim to minimize vulnerability to disaster in a population, to avoid (prevention) or to limit (mitigation and preparedness) the adverse impacts of hazards, within the broad context of sustainable development.

Introduction

Disasters are often described as a result of the combination of: the exposure to a hazard; the conditions of vulnerability that are present; and insufficient capacity or measures to reduce or cope with the potential negative consequences. Disaster impacts may include loss of life, injury, disease and other negative effects on human physical, mental and social wellbeing, together with damage to property, destruction of assets, loss of services, social and economic disruption and environmental degradation.

(UNISDR 2007)

Disasters, emergencies, and other crises may cause ill health directly or through the disruption of health systems, facilities and services, leaving many without access to health care in times of emergency. They also affect critical infrastructure such as water and energy supplies, sanitation systems and safe shelter, which are essential for health (see Chapters 5, 6 and 9). Disasters can also impede progress on development gains in health and other sectors (see Chapter 3).

Public health professionals have a role in the response to disasters but must also work with other agencies in disaster preparedness. Health protection and wider public health and disaster risk management are considered to be closely linked and largely synonymous (Murray et. al. 2012). The systematic analysis and management of health risks posed by emergencies and disasters should include: prevention of hazards; vulnerability reduction to prevent and mitigate risks; preparedness; early warning and detection; and analysis of disaster trends, response and recovery and evaluation.

The impact of a disaster on health can be mitigated through effective planning (disaster preparedness) and subsequent implementation of the planned response. Disaster preparedness and response are often undertaken by local agencies in partnership with national and international organizations. International guidance exists which aims to build resilience of nations and communities to disasters (UNISDR 2005, 2015), such as the International Health Regulations (WHO 2005) and the Sendai Framework for Action 2015–2030 (see Chapter 14). Public health professionals should support these international processes, ensuring as far as possible their local implementation.

Types of disaster

Disasters can be classified as natural, biological, technological or societal (WHO/UNISDR/HPA 2011).

- *Natural disasters* include both geological hazards (earthquakes, volcanoes) and hydro-meteorological hazards (wind storms, floods). The incidence of some natural disasters has been increasing (this is discussed in more detail below).
- *Technological disasters* are those caused by human activities, and include explosions, chemical releases, and major transport accidents.
- *Biological disasters* are major outbreaks caused by new and re-emerging infectious diseases such as Ebola, Zika, SARS, influenza (H1N1 and H5N1) and cholera. Biological emergencies have assumed an increasing importance in the last few decades.
- *Societal disasters* or 'complex emergencies' often include violent conflict (such as civil war) but may also be associated with natural hazards such as floods or drought. Such events can cause displacement of people both within and across borders. It is often difficult to categorize the 'type' of event when there is a complex emergency.

Table 10.1 describes the global frequency of disasters by disaster type and by region, for natural and technological disasters. Floods are the most common type of disaster. Asia is the region most affected by natural and technological disasters. Categorization of the type of disaster can be difficult. For example, there are several different causes of flooding which are not described in EM-DAT. A disaster might also be associated with several hazards. For example, in 2011, Japan experienced a tsunami, an earthquake and a technological disaster (incident at a nuclear power station).

Impacts of disasters

Disasters can have a long-term impact on the national economy. Economic impacts include: loss of exports; loss of tourist trade; diversion of national funds for clean-up, reconstruction and disaster relief (Hochrainer 2009).

It is often difficult to get accurate information on the impacts of disasters, particularly in low-income countries. The Centre for Research on the Epidemiology of Disasters (CRED) has a global dataset on all types of disasters (EM-DAT). Various definitions of disasters exist, but the one used

Table 10.1 Total number of disaster events 2002–11

Disaster type	Africa	Americas	Asia	Europe	Oceania	Total
Drought/famine	126	50	48	10	3	237
Earthquake/tsunami	23	39	181	33	13	289
Extreme temperatures	3	41	60	130	1	235
Flood	450	368	690	237	48	1793
Forest/scrub fire	10	47	14	34	9	114
Insect infestation	13	n.d.r.	n.d.r.	n.d.r.	1	14
Mass movement (including landslides, mud slides, rockfalls, avalanches, etc.)	14	42	124	10	7	197
Volcanic eruption	6	24	21	1	10	62
Windstorms (including tropical cyclones, tornadoes)	89	336	386	146	65	1,022
Total natural disasters	**734**	**947**	**1,524**	**601**	**157**	**3,963**

Source: Data from EM_DAT disaster database, adapted from Table 9 of IFRC (2012)

Note: Number of events may not add up due to recording issues (see the following comments about problems with accurate categorization for the EM-DAT); n.d.r. = no data recorded

by EM-DAT is an event where 10 or more people are killed, or 100 or more people affected, or there is a declaration of a state of emergency, or call for international assistance (CRED 2012).

Robust information on the impacts of disasters is needed to improve the disaster response, and for global action. There are several reasons why it can be difficult to get accurate information on disasters, including:

- Enumerating disaster events and impacts will depend on the information sources used. In the past, only the more significant events were likely to be recorded, making a proper analysis of trends in disasters unreliable.
- Disaster statistics typically only immediately reported total deaths. Useful information on mortality, such as cause or age, is not available. Information on non-fatal impacts from disasters is also not usually available in global datasets. Further, only the immediate effects on mortality are included, not any longer-term indirect consequences.

Many consequences of a disaster can be avoided by good response planning and by ensuring resilience of the physical infrastructure. The consequences of disasters are dependent on social and economic factors, for example, failure to adhere to building codes in earthquake zones, poor management of flood barriers, lack of management of disaster coordination centres or failure to implement early warning systems. The health effects of disasters will also depend on the capacity of individuals and households to cope with the hazard.

Health impacts of disasters

In the following sections we explore the health impacts of natural disasters and technological disasters.

Health impacts of natural disasters

This section describes what is currently known about the health effects of natural disasters from epidemiological and other observational studies. Disasters tend to occur over a short period of time and may involve many deaths and injuries.

Hydro-meteorological events (tropical cyclones, floods) occur more frequently than geological disasters such as earthquakes, volcanic eruptions and tsunamis (Table 10.1). However, earthquakes have a bigger impact in terms of numbers of deaths (both per event and total disaster-attributable mortality). Different disaster types have different regional distributions. The impact of natural disasters is not equally distributed due to differences in socioeconomic factors (the capacity to respond) and geography (e.g. tropical cyclones only occur in certain regions and the distribution of earthquakes is determined by the activity of tectonic plates). Some regions are much more vulnerable to certain types of natural hazard, for example over 90 per cent of deaths due to tropical cyclones occur in Asia.

Health effects of floods

The impact of a flood disaster can affect health in several ways (Ahern et al. 2005), and at various phases (see Table 10.2). The initial floodwaters may cause drowning and trauma. After the onset of floodwaters, there is a risk of infectious diseases linked to drinking contaminated water and the interruption of sewerage and waste disposal systems. The psychological impacts caused by natural disasters can also be significant. Public health problems can also occur due to large-scale displacement of populations, especially if in temporary settlements.

Health effects of geological hazards

Geological disasters, such as earthquakes and volcanoes, are more likely to involve death and severe injury than flood events. Figure 10.1 describes the main factors that determine the health impacts of geological hazards. Individual factors that determine vulnerability include age and gender, although the age groups most at risk from death and injury were found to vary from event to event in a review (Ramirez and Peek-Asa 2005). Building construction – whether the building collapses – is a key determinant of mortality and injuries from earthquakes.

Table 10.2 The health effects of flooding

Impacts on health	Pre-onset phase	Onset phase	Post-onset phase
Direct	• Injuries	• Death (drowning) • Injuries (e.g. cuts, abrasions, sprains, fractures, punctures)	• Faecal-oral and other diarrhoeal disease • Vector- and rodent-borne disease (e.g. malaria, leptospirosis) • Respiratory infections • Skin/eye infections • Mental health • Snake bites
Indirect	–	Health outcomes associated with: • Damage to health care infrastructure, and loss of essential drugs • Chemical contamination of food and water stocks • Damage to water and sanitation infrastructure • Damage to crops and/or disruption of food supplies • Damage/destruction of property (e.g. lack of shelter may lead to increased exposure to disease vectors) • Population displacement	

Source: Adapted from Ahern et al. (2005)

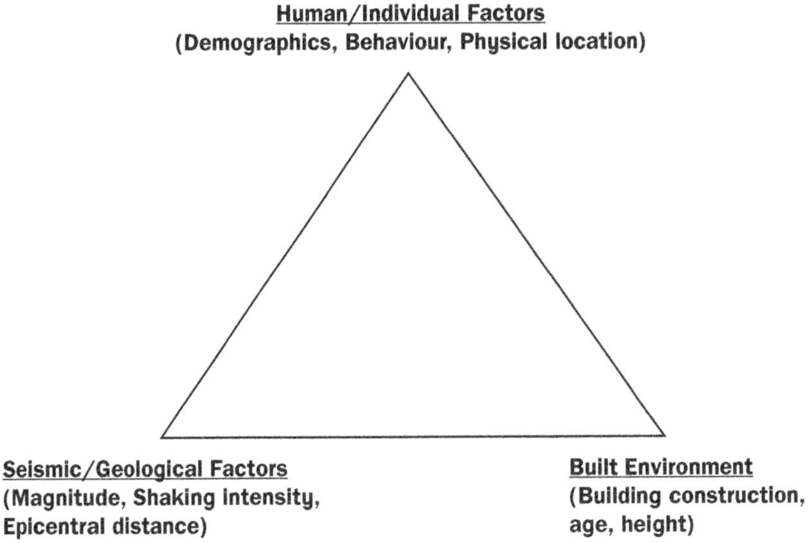

Human/Individual Factors
(Demographics, Behaviour, Physical location)

Seismic/Geological Factors
(Magnitude, Shaking intensity, Epicentral distance)

Built Environment
(Building construction, age, height)

Figure 10.1 The epidemiological triangle.
Source: Ramirez and Peek-Asa (2005).

Activity 10.1

Disasters can have different effects on different groups, depending on social or physiological vulnerability. Read the extract below. Which population sub-groups may have been most affected by the tsunami? How would you investigate this?

Case study: Southeast Asia Tsunami 2004

On December the 26th 2004 a series of earthquakes with epicentres off of Northern Sumatra (Aceh) in Indonesia and the resultant tsunamis hit Southeast Asia causing serious damage and loss of life. The earthquake measured 9 on the Richter scale, one of the largest earthquakes in the last 40 years. The initial priorities were to ensure clean water, adequate shelter, food, sanitation and healthcare for the 3–5 million people affected, and to identify and bury thousands of bodies. A week after the disaster there was widespread shortage of clean water and a risk of disease outbreaks. Health education received a high priority in India and Sri Lanka to help prevent the spread of disease. Providing health services to displaced people was a significant challenge. Six weeks after the disaster, the second phase of the post-disaster health programme was in place and the focus was on rebuilding infrastructure, increasing capacity and assessing and rehabilitating local health systems. The mental health and nutritional status of many tsunami survivors was still of serious concern. . .

The worst affected area was Aceh on the island of Sumatra in Indonesia; more than 70% of the inhabitants of some coastal villages are reported to have died. The exact number of victims has not been documented whilst the number of homeless was estimated at 800,000. After the disaster more than 100 aid organisations and UN agencies were operating in Indonesia. Other agencies provided emergency food, water, medical care and shelter to about 330,000 people and assisted in constructing temporary settlements for 150,000 families.

Indonesia was hardest hit in terms of loss of life and physical damage, but seems to have escaped the worst of the tsunami's economic disruption. In the year following the 2004 tsunami, the Indonesian economy nevertheless recorded its strongest growth since the Asian financial crisis in the 1990s. . . The main affected area, Aceh, is rich in resources but far from crucial to overall output. The World Bank Country Assistance Strategy (2009–2012) "Investing in Indonesia's

Institutions" places high emphasis on reducing Indonesia's vulnerability to natural disasters and disaster risks management as a core work program. . . After the 2004 tsunami, Indonesia enacted a new Law on Disaster Management, although implementation remains a major challenge. This is the first priority of the Hyogo Framework for Action (HFA). In addition, a new National Disaster Management Agency (BNPB) has been created and Indonesia has now formulated the first three-year National Action Plan (2010–2012) for Disaster Risk Reduction.

(GFDRR 2010)

Feedback

Several groups may have been more affected by the disaster.

- Children, especially those under the age of 5 are particularly vulnerable to disaster. They are more likely to be injured, lost, unable to access help or health care, or exposed to greater danger through separation from their families or carers.
- Older persons or persons with disabilities are also more vulnerable. Older people are more likely to have a chronic illness or disability that limits their daily activities.
- For some types of disaster, women suffer disproportionately. In any emergency, up to 20 per cent of affected women of childbearing age are likely to be pregnant.
- Low-income households may have been more vulnerable to the disaster, particularly after the event, as they lacked the capacity to cope.
- Indigenous groups may also be vulnerable as they may have less access to government resources or health care.

How could you investigate the effects by sub-group?

- Quantitative analysis. Collect information on deaths or hospital admissions from the disaster by age group, gender, etc. and cause of death.
- Qualitative information. Interview survivors about impacts and access to support after the disasters. Interview public health professionals or NGOs/civil society who were involved in the humanitarian response.

Health impacts of technological disasters

Technological disasters cause a range of health impacts in the local populations, and can also cause long-term damage to the local environment. Table 10.3 describes the major technological disasters (industrial and transport accidents) that have occurred in the last two decades. These have had a range of causes from explosions in munitions and firework factories to ingestion of contaminated medicines and foods. The causes of technological disasters emphasize the need for effective planning and the enforcement of industrial and transport safety regulations.

A chemical incident is the unexpected release into the environment of a substance that is (potentially) hazardous to humans. Chemical releases arise from technological incidents, impact of natural hazards, or from conflict and terrorism. A description of a chemical disaster (Seveso disaster) in which the accidental release of a toxic chemical (dioxin) had serious implications for health is explored in Chapter 4 (Activity 4.4). There can also be long-term effects from chemical exposures, such as dioxins, that need to be taken into account and carefully monitored over years or decades after the disaster event (Svendsen et al. 2012). The case study below describes one of the worst ever industrial accidents – the chemical release in Bhopal, India, in 1984.

Table 10.3 Transport and industrial disasters with greatest mortality in period 1994–2012

Industrial accidents			Transport accidents		
Country	Date	No. killed	Country	Date	No. killed
Nigeria, explosion	17/10/1998	1,082	Senegal, water	26/09/2002	1,200
Nigeria, explosion	26/12/2006	269	Egypt, water	02/02/2006	1,028
Nigeria, explosion	10/07/2000	260	Estonia, water	28/09/1994	912
Pakistan, fire	11/09/2012	240	Tanzania Uni Rep, water	21/05/1996	869
China P Rep, explosion	23/12/2003	234	Philippines, water	21/06/2008	815
China P Rep, explosion	14/02/2005	214	Bangladesh, water	08/07/2003	528
China P Rep, other	17/07/2001	200	Indonesia, water	29/06/2000	481
Nigeria, poisoning	January 2010	200	Congo Dem Rep, air	08/01/1996	422
Nigeria, explosion	13/05/2006	175	Haiti, water	08/09/1997	400
China P Rep, other	18/08/2007	172	Indonesia, water	30/12/2006	400

Source: EMDAT

**Box 10.1:   Case study: accidental release of methyl-
                      isocyanate in Bhopal, India, 1984**

On 3 December 1984, an accidental release at night of 40 tons of methyl-
isocyanate gas from a pesticide plant in Bhopal, India, into the atmosphere
killed at least 3,800 people acutely and caused significant morbidity and
premature death for many thousands more (Broughton 2005). It is now
believed that over 20,000 people have died from exposure to the gas since
the accident, and there are 120,000 chronically ill survivors. This incident
illustrated some of the problems associated with a lack of planning for
disasters. It occurred in a developing country where industrial practices
may not be as rigorously controlled as in developed countries. There was
public housing beside the plant; the release occurred at night, making it
more difficult to alert the nearby residents so there was an additional delay
in warning them; there were only limited medical facilities nearby and there
was little understanding of the toxic nature of the leak.

The company who owned and operated the site immediately tried to
dissociate itself from legal responsibility although it was later reported
that key safety equipment designed to stop the escape of the gas was
not functioning or was turned off. Eventually the company reached a
settlement with the Indian government through mediation of that country's Supreme Court, accepted responsibility and paid $470 million in
compensation. This was a relatively small amount based on significant
underestimations of the long-term health consequences of exposure and
the number of people exposed (Broughton 2005). There remain weak
regulations in many countries controlling the siting of potentially high-risk
industries and insufficient emergency planning for chemical disasters.
Many lessons were identified including:

- industry and government need to give proper financial support to
  local communities so they can provide medical and other necessary
  services to reduce morbidity, mortality and material loss in the aftermath
  of industrial accidents;
- local governments must not allow high-risk industrial facilities to be
  situated within urban areas, regardless of the evolution of land use
  over time;
- the need for enforceable international standards for environmental
  safety, with preventative strategies to avoid similar accidents;
- the need for industrial disaster preparedness.

Clear, concise contingency plans are needed to prevent or reduce the
effects of technological disasters. There should first be an assessment of
the likely hazards and their potential to cause adverse health effects (see
section on health impact assessment of chemical hazards in Chapter 4).

This hazard assessment will help to inform the response plans to mitigate risks and reduce health and other impacts.

Disaster management

Disaster preparedness

Disaster preparedness is the term used to describe all the activities and measures that can be taken in advance of a disaster to promote an effective response and so limit impacts. These activities include the issuance of timely and effective early warnings of disasters. Depending on the type of disaster this may be minutes, hours or days. Another important action is to have a plan for the temporary evacuation of people from threatened locations.

A pre-existing emergency public health plan is key to an effective flexible and appropriate response. Immediate consequences of a disaster may occur from lack of food and water, or access to sanitation, as well as the risk of chemical contamination. The provision of safe water for drinking, washing and domestic activities is a public health priority, as well as the safe removal of waste (toilets and waste disposal), together with health promotion activities to encourage protective healthy behavioural practices among the affected population.

✏ Activity 10.2

Hurricane Sandy made landfall on Haiti in October 2012. Read the extract from the news report from the WHO below. You are a representative from the WHO and have just arrived. What are the public health response issues you need to address?

Report from Friday 2 November 2012

Some 1.8 million Haitians have been affected by Hurricane Sandy, the United Nations relief agency said today after its first assessment of the situation in the region, adding that food security remains an urgent concern in the Caribbean nation. Initial data collected by the UN Office for the Coordination of Humanitarian Affairs (OCHA) showed Hurricane Sandy, which ploughed through the Caribbean country before hitting the eastern coast of the United States, killed 60 people and significantly damaged critical infrastructure such as roads, schools and hospitals in addition to destroying thousands of homes.

It was reported that for the past 5 days, "Floodwater had been receding since Sunday but more than 18,000 homes have been flooded, damaged or destroyed," and that food security remains a main concern as the country is now struggling with the combined impact of hurricanes Sandy and Isaac, which hit in August, as well as drought. Preliminary data estimated that food security had been severely affected, with up to 2 million people at risk of malnutrition. In addition to food insecurity, OCHA said it is concerned about the nearly 350,000 people that are still living in camps for internally displaced persons (IDPs) as a result of a devastating earthquake which hit the country in January 2010. While most vulnerable IDPs in camps that had been evacuated before the storm have returned home, some 1,500 people remain in 15 hurricane shelters.

During the same briefing, a spokesperson for the UN World Health Organization (WHO) reported that access to health services and restocking basic supplies was limited as rivers had become impassable and roads had been obstructed. It also warned that poor sanitary conditions could increase the risk of water-borne diseases such as cholera, which is still endemic in the country.

The WHO spokesperson said there has already been an increase in cholera alerts, especially in the south, and added that field teams are monitoring the situation closely. WHO is also working with the Government in the area to ensure that health supplies could be delivered to treatment centres that had been damaged by strong winds and flooding, he added.

(UN 2012)

Feedback

Using your public health skills you will also have considered some or all of the following to respond to the Haiti hurricane.

- Determine, by working in partnership with Haiti's Ministry of Health, the needs and the programme for response including what UN agencies and international NGOs can best contribute.
- Determine how best to use field hospitals.
- Determine, in conjunction with the Ministry of Health and local needs assessment, if an immunization progamme is required.
- Determine where to undertake epidemiological surveillance to provide appropriate and useful rapid needs assessments to focus response more effectively.
- Evaluate the response, and identify lessons to build into updating and exercising the local health emergency plan.
- Publish your findings in an open peer review journal to ensure others can learn from the findings to improve their own responses (guidance on how to write such a report is available in Kulling et al. 2011).

Emergency response and planning for disasters

The two main types of emergency plan are as follows.

- *National or regional plans:* these define responsibilities and procedures for key personnel in emergency response organizations, public health and environmental departments and should include plans for coordination of civil defence organizations and the voluntary sector.
- *Local plan – detailed plans:* identifying as far as possible local hazards and addressing the risks as fully as possible. Also including lists of individuals and organizations involved with associated specific responsibilities.

The stages of the disaster management cycle are illustrated in Figure 10.2 and are summarized below and in the next activity (WHO 2009):

- *Prevention:* reducing the potential effects of disasters by preparation and good planning. This includes ensuring there is adequate physical infrastructure, and measures to ensure continuity of transport systems, water supplies and waste removal, and water supplies for fire-fighting in

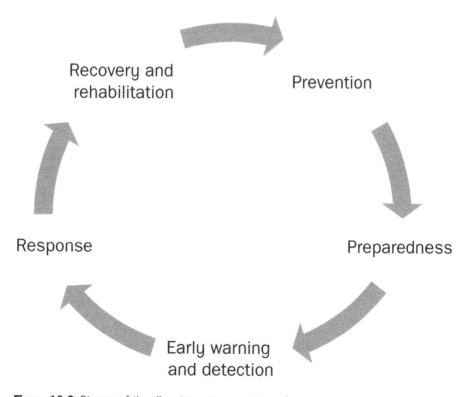

Figure 10.2 Stages of the disaster management cycle.

rural and urban areas. Replacing industrial materials with less toxic or less flammable chemicals, reducing the amount of stored chemicals, building in technical safety measures, land use planning to ensure that facilities are located where a release would not harm the public.

- *Preparedness:* includes the anticipation of disasters likely to occur; understanding the organization of personnel and services; coordination, location and inventory of supplies and equipment; review of all community and industrial facilities and their vulnerability to disaster; review and learning from disaster scenarios. Preparation for the general public may include guidance on how to build a disaster supplies kit to ensure that if evacuation is required all relevant supplies including medication can be taken (FEMA 2012.)

- *Warning or alerting phase (if the disaster can be forecast in a timely way):* includes advance warning for some disasters, particularly natural events such as floods, windstorms and cyclones. Warnings can also permit emergency services to assemble, and for timely, appropriate information to be provided for the public via mass media. For example, communities may be advised to evacuate their homes if they live in the path of a flood or a wildfire. Technical alerting systems such as gas or radiation detection equipment can be used to monitor for a release within or near a facility.

- *Response:* the first step is to assess the extent of a disaster and, where possible, limit its impact by using emergency plans to respond including – if a chemical incident – terminating a release, preventing spread of contamination and providing advice to the public (WHO 2009). Other public health steps include:
  - activating the disaster/incident emergency plan, including a public health response;
  - providing an initial assessment and advising and alerting health care services;
  - ensuring coordination and integration of the public health response;
  - conducting a best outcome assessment for both immediate and long-term actions;
  - disseminating information and advice to responders, the public and the media;
  - registering all exposed individuals and collecting samples to eliminate exposure;
  - conducting acute and longer-term needs assessments and investigations;
  - documenting all information for further investigations.

- *Recovery/rehabilitation:* requires health outcome assessment during or immediately after the incident to assess the impacts from the disaster. This involves obtaining data on those exposed and documenting their potential health effects from the disaster as well as psychosocial-related effects such as anxiety and stress. Data should be collected on both morbidity and mortality outcomes.

Activity 10.3

The path of hurricanes (tropical cyclones) is tracked for some time before they make landfall. This allows some time (from hours to days) to prepare for the disaster. Design a hurricane disaster management plan for a tropical island in the Pacific Ocean. Refer to the example of the hurricane in Haiti described earlier in the chapter for some ideas.

Feedback

Your response should include a range of action under the four phases:

- preparedness phase;
- warning and alerting phase;
- response phase;
- recovery/rehabilitation phase.

The actions should be appropriate to the context. Your plan could also include:

- data collection in order to gain information on the health impacts of the disaster;
- evaluation and monitoring in order to learn what has been effective.

Changing pressures and trends in disasters

Trends in disasters indicate that, overall, populations are becoming less vulnerable to natural and technological hazards. However, the mortality impact of some disasters, such as flooding, is increasing due to population growth (Kundzewicz et al. 2014). Furthermore, there remain large differences in vulnerability between countries. For example, a study by UNISDR estimated that the mortality risk from disasters was 225 times greater in low-income countries than in high-income countries (UNISDR 2011). Decreases in the mortality impacts of disasters are due to improvements in early warning measures as well as disaster risk reduction measures.

Population growth in disaster-prone areas, particularly urbanization in coastal areas, has been a major cause of the increased number of flood events. The concentration of people and property in flood zones has been well documented, particularly in Asia (Quarantelli 2003). Further, there is evidence that mortality risk from disaster increases with economic development, before it then decreases (Patt et al. 2010). This may be due to rapid urbanization increasing vulnerability to disasters before the benefits of economic development and increased regulation take effect.

Several key factors have been identified that affect future disaster risks (Foresight 2012). These include population growth and urbanization in disaster risk areas. Global changes will have both positive and negative effects and are summarized in Table 10.4. The social and economic determinants of vulnerability are extremely important. Good governance is essential in order to ensure that safety standards and preparedness actions are implemented.

Some types of weather-related disasters are expected to increase in frequency and intensity as a result of global climate change (IPCC 2012) (see Chapter 12). These include heatwaves and coastal flooding (where coastal defences are not upgraded). River flooding may also increase in some areas due to climate change but such projections are very uncertain.

Ecosystem degradation can also increase the risk of disasters. Many natural environments provide protection against flooding (hazard control). For example, mangroves have been shown to reduce the impact of storm surges in coastal populations (Das and Vincent 2009). A systematic review of the benefits of salt marshes found that that this ecosystem reduced the impacts of coastal hazards (Shepard et al. 2011). It is therefore important to maintain the ecosystem service of hazard control to protect populations from disasters (see Chapter 13).

Table 10.4 Summary of trends and potential impacts of eight key drivers on the components of future disaster risk

Driver	Effect on exposure	Effect on vulnerability	Effect on resilience	Uncertainties in future trends
Global environmental change	↑	↑	↓	Low: environmental trends are likely to continue even if concerted policy action is taken now. Out to 2040, the overall trend is largely predetermined by actions already taken and the current state of the environment.
Demographic change	↑	↑	↓	Low: much of the future age distribution is already determined by the current distribution.
Conflict and instability	↑	↑	↓	Medium: the specific nature of future wars is very uncertain. However, a large reduction in conflict seems unlikely, as does a return to large-scale interstate war. Civil unrest and instability will continue to flare up unpredictably.
Political and governance change	X	↑	↑ ↓	High: there is no certainty that democratization will continue or whether it will lead to increased participation in

(continued)

Table 10.4 (Continued)

Driver	Effect on exposure	Effect on vulnerability	Effect on resilience	Uncertainties in future trends
				government processes. International aid and development regimes will continue to change.
Urbanization	↟	↟	↟ ↓	Low: continued urbanization seems likely, although the rate may slow.
Economic growth	↟	↟	↟ ↓	High: future global economic crises could change the balance of contemporary economic powers, composition of financial regulatory regimes or the structure of global institutions.
Globalization	↟	↟	↟ ↓	Medium: economically and politically, the world in the future will likely be a more connected place, with pockets of isolation remaining for geographical or political reasons. As connectivity expands, accountability and flows of knowledge may increase.
Technological change	X	↑ ↓	↟ ↓	Medium: the most important technological innovations are likely to be those not yet conceived, and attitudes to new technologies are difficult to predict. However, overall spread of new technologies is likely to continue.

X The dominant effect of the driver on the determinant of risk is negligible
↟ The driver can lead to a significant increase in the determinant of risk
↑ The driver can lead to a slight increase in the determinant of risk
↓ The driver can lead to a significant decrease in the determinant of risk
↓ The driver can lead to a slight decrease in the determinant of risk
Source: Foresight (2012)

Summary

The health, environmental and economic costs of natural and technological disasters are immense. We have explored some of the issues associated with the stages of the disaster management cycle: prevention, prepared-ness, early warning and detection, response and recovery. Planning for disaster prevention and relief is essential in order to minimize the impacts of disasters. Strengthening and integrating public health and disaster management measures will increase the resilience of those at risk.

References

Ahern, M., Kovats, R.S., Wilkinson, P., Few, R. and Matthies, F. (2005) Global health impacts of floods: epidemiologic evidence, *Epidemiologic Reviews*, 27: 36–46.

Broughton, E. (2005) The Bhopal disaster and its aftermath: a review, *Environmental Health*, 4: 6.

CRED (2012) *Emergency Events Database (EM-DAT)*, http://www.emdat.be/, accessed 11 March 2012.

Das, S. and Vincent, J.R. (2009) Mangroves protected villages and reduced death toll during Indian super cyclone, *Proceedings of the National Academy of Sciences USA*, 106: 7357–60.

FEMA (Federal Emergency Management Agency) (2012) Build a kit, http://www.ready.gov/build-a-kit, accessed 4 November 2012.

Foresight (2012) *Reducing Risks of Future Disasters. Priorities for Decision Makers. Final Project Report.* London: The Government Office for Science.

GFDRR (Global Facility for Disaster Reduction and Recovery) (2010) *Country Programming Framework: Indonesia*, http://gfdrr.org/ctryprogram_pdfs/id.pdf, accessed 4 November 2012.

Hochrainer, S. (2009) Assessing the macroeconomic impacts of natural disasters: are there any? Policy Research Working Paper 4968. New York: The World Bank Sustainable Development Network Vice Presidency, Global Facility for Disaster Reduction and Recovery Unit.

IFRC (International Federation of Red Cross and Red Crescent Societies) (2012) *World Disasters Report 2012*, http://www.ifrc.org/PageFiles/99703/1216800-WDR%202012-EN-LR.pdf, accessed 3 November 2012.

IPCC (2012) *Managing the Risks of Extreme Events and Disasters to Advance Climate Change Adaptation. A Special Report of Working Groups I and II of the Intergovernmental Panel on Climate Change* (Field, C.B. et al. eds), p. 582. Cambridge: Cambridge University Press.

Kulling, P., Birnbaum, M., Murray, V. and Rockenschaub, G. (2011) Guidelines for reports on health crises and critical health events – a tool for the development of disaster medicine research, *Prehospital and Disaster Medicine*, 26: s17.

Kundzewicz, Z.W., Kanae, S., Seneviratne, S.I. et al. (2014) Flood risk and climate change: global and regional perspectives, *Hydrological Sciences Journal*, 59(1): 1–28.

Murray, V., McBean, G., Bhatt, M. et al. (2012) Case studies, in Field, C.B. et al. (eds) *Managing the Risks of Extreme Events and Disasters to Advance Climate Change Adaptation*. A Special Report of Working Groups I and II of the Intergovernmental Panel on Climate Change (IPCC), pp. 487–542. Cambridge: Cambridge University Press.

Patt, A.G., Tadross, M., Nussbaumer, P. et al. (2010) Estimating least-developed countries' vulnerability to climate-related extreme events over the next 50 years, *Proceedings of the National Academy of Sciences USA*, 107: 1333–7.

Quarantelli, E.L. (2003) *Urban vulnerability to disasters in developing countries: managing risks*, in A. Kreimer et al. (eds) *Building Safer Cities: The future of disaster risk.* Washington, DC: World Bank.

Ramirez, M. and Peek-Asa, C. (2005) Epidemiology of traumatic injuries from earthquakes, *Epidemiological Review*, 27: 47–55.

Shepard, C.C., Crain, C.M. and Beck, M.W. (2011) The protective role of coastal marshes: a systematic review and meta-analysis, *PLoS One*, 6(11): e27374, doi: 10.1371/journal.pone.0027374.

Svendsen, E.R., Runkle, J.R., Dhara, V.R. et al. (2012) Epidemiologic methods: lessons learned from environmental public health disasters – Chernobyl, the World Trade Center, Bhopal, and Graniteville, South Carolina, *International Journal of Environmental Research and Public Health*, 9(8): 2894–909.

UN (2012) UN News Centre (2012) UN relief agency estimates 1.8 million Haitians have been affected by Hurricane Sandy, http://www.un.org/apps/news/story.asp?NewsID=43405#.VySABUavwWo, accessed 11 April 2013.

UNISDR (2005) *Hyogo Framework for Action 2005–2015, ISDR International Strategy for Disaster Reduction: building the resilience of nations and communities to disasters*. Geneva: UNISDR.

UNISDR (2007) Terminology, http://www.unisdr.org/we/inform/terminology, accessed 13 October 2012.

UNISDR (2011) *GAR 2011 – Revealing Risk, Redefining Development*. Geneva: UN International Stratety for Disaster Reduction.

UNISDR (2015) *Sendai Framework for Disaster Risk Reduction 2015–2030*. Geneva: UN International Stratety for Disaster Reduction.

WHO (2005) *International Health Regulations*, 2nd edn, http://whqlibdoc.who.int/publications/2008/9789241580410_eng.pdf, accessed 13 October 2012.

WHO (2009) *Manual for the Public Health Management of Chemical Incidents*, http://www.who.int/environmental_health_emergencies/publications/FINAL-PHM-Chemical-Incidents_web.pdf, accessed 15 September 2012

WHO/UNISDR/HPA (2011) *Disaster Risk Management for Health*. Geneva: WHO, http://www.who.int/hac/events/disaster_reduction_2011/en/.

11 Energy

Noah Scovronick

Overview

Energy is essential for human activity. The demand for energy also increases with population growth and economic development. A consistent supply of energy offers many benefits, including household energy for cooking and heating and the ability to provide modern health care. Not all populations have equal access to energy; high-income countries use much more and much cleaner energy than low-income countries, and energy-related health impacts can differ substantially between populations. Currently, the world depends on energy from fossil fuels, but there is a trend towards cleaner and renewable energy sources.

Learning objectives

By the end of this chapter you will be able to:

- describe the health effects associated with different forms of power (energy) generation and distribution
- describe the linkages between energy efficiency and health
- appraise methods for quantifying the health impacts associated with specific energy scenarios or policies
- evaluate how health impacts can be used in energy policy decision-making

Key terms

Co-benefits (also called ancillary benefits): Benefits to health that may accrue from policies or programmes implemented for other (non-health) reasons.

Energy efficiency: The ability to use less energy while providing the same product or service. This differs from the definition in the housing chapter. The definition here is more qualitative and a relative definition for energy services.

Energy ladder: A model of household energy use whereby increasing income is associated with cleaner and more efficient energy sources (movement up the energy ladder).

Energy poverty: The condition of having inadequate access to energy, namely lack of household access to electricity and lack of clean cooking fuel.

Life-cycle analysis: An assessment approach that ensures that all stages in a fuel's life cycle are considered, sometimes called a 'cradle to grave' approach.

Renewable energy: Energy sources that do not deplete, or are naturally replenished after use.

Introduction

'Energy' can be defined as the ability to do work. At its most basic, we require energy in the form of food to perform essential metabolic functions. But we also rely on other forms of energy inputs in almost all areas of life that affect our health and wellbeing, from cooking and keeping warm to providing the electricity necessary for our hospitals to function (Activity 11.1).

 Activity 11.1

Think about the energy you use in your everyday life and note down the reasons you use it, and if known, its source.

Feedback

People have many different energy requirements, and you will have noted some of the following:

- basic human needs – heating, lighting, cooking (using electricity, oil, gas, biomass fuel);
- agriculture – irrigation, mechanization (using wind, oil, electricity, water);
- urban living – basic services for city life (using oil, electricity, coal);
- transport (using oil, physical energy – walking/cycling, electricity);
- industry (using electricity, oil, coal, wind, water).

Electricity production still relies largely on fossil fuel sources, with smaller proportions from hydroelectric production and nuclear power. Electricity from renewable sources other than hydroelectricity is a small but growing proportion of global electricity production.

There are many different energy sources available for human use. The vast majority of energy used to provide energy services (mechanical work and heat) derives from the sun: fossil fuels, biomass, and, to a lesser extent, direct capture of solar energy through solar-thermal and photovoltaic systems. Fossil fuels include coal, petroleum (oil) and natural gas, which have been formed over millions of years from organic matter. Other sources of energy include wind and wave power, hydropower nuclear fission and geothermal energy (which is mainly derived from natural processes inside the Earth's core and crust).

Fuel is defined as 'material such as coal, gas, or oil that is burned to produce heat or power' (*Oxford English Dictionary*) or fissionable material that produces heat as a byproduct of radioactive decay. An ideal fuel source for producing energy for human needs is one which is:

- energy-dense (lots of energy per unit volume);
- light (for transporting);
- stable and safe to store and transport;
- abundant;
- clean (produces few toxic byproducts/pollutants);
- cost-effective to extract or produce.

The choice of fuel or energy source for a given activity depends on many factors including its end-use, social acceptability, and on the population that could be exposed to pollutants. Most countries have a diverse energy matrix (their energy is produced from multiple sources), which usually is heavily influenced by the availability of local energy sources.

Energy: production and use

The abundant energy resources provided by fossil fuels have enabled unprecedented economic growth and technological development, which has been accompanied by increases in human health and wellbeing. However, this energy transition has not reached everybody equally. There are also large disparities in energy use: high-income countries consume 13 times more energy per person than low-income countries, while the difference is over 100-fold between the richest and poorest populations.

Fossil fuels are very convenient, possessing many of the desirable qualities for an energy source (see above). Most high-income countries have
depended on them for their economic development, and they still comprise
the majority of the world's energy supply.

Burning fossil fuels causes indoor and outdoor air pollution (see Chapters
6 and 7) and releases greenhouse gases (GHGs) which cause climate
change (see Chapter 12). Ensuring their continued supply can also contribute to geopolitical tensions and even conflict, as fossil fuel reserves are
concentrated in a relatively small number of exporting countries. Further,
fossil fuels are non-renewable energy sources, meaning they are not
replenished after they are burned – at least not on a human timescale.

Many countries are trying to reduce their dependence on fossil fuels by
shifting towards renewable energy sources. Combined with increased
energy efficiency, the use of renewables has the potential to provide a
sustainable supply of energy without the negative consequences of air
pollution and climate change. The proportion and type of renewable
energy in the energy matrix varies substantially from country to country
(see Figure 11.1). For example, Brazil, with huge freshwater resources, is
the only country with substantial hydroelectricity use, while Saudi Arabia's
energy supply reflects its immense oil and gas reserves.

The energy matrix is an important factor in determining a country's environmental quality, and different energy sources affect health in different
ways, as discussed in the next section.

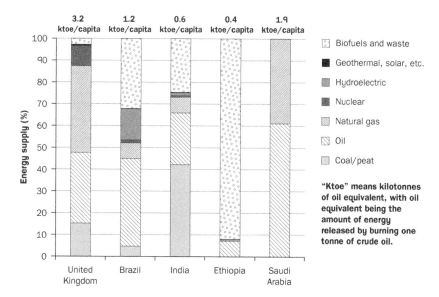

Figure 11.1 Total energy supply in select countries, 2009 – excludes trade in
electricity.

Source: IEA (2012).

Health impacts of different energy types

At an international level, the amount of energy consumed is strongly correlated with health up to around 1,500 kg of oil equivalent per person per
year (see Figure 11.2). Above that level, the relationship with life expectancy or infant mortality, for example, is fairly flat – indicating that increasing per capita energy use is not necessarily accompanied by further gain in
health. High energy use is an accompaniment of socioeconomic development in general, and many factors may account for improved health in the
more advanced economies. Nonetheless, access to plentiful and affordable
energy provides multiple services that can contribute to health, ranging
from protection against heat and cold, to enabling the functioning of
advanced health care services (and allowing us to access them via transportation). Insufficient access to energy prevents large segments of the world's
populations from enjoying these benefits.

Energy production and access to energy services may also have negative
impacts on human health, through air pollution and by encouraging unhealthy
lifestyles including sub-optimal levels of physical activity and supporting the
production, distribution and consumption of energy-dense processed foods
that contribute to excess food energy intake and poor dietary patterns more
generally. Because energy use is strongly related to income, populations at
different levels of economic development will be exposed to different environmental hazards. The concept of the energy ladder illustrates this (see
Figure 11.3). In general, richer populations tend to use more and cleaner
energy, and are more likely to separate production from end-use.

The following activity explores the use of natural experiments to investigate
health impacts that result from a change in the environment. Epidemiologists

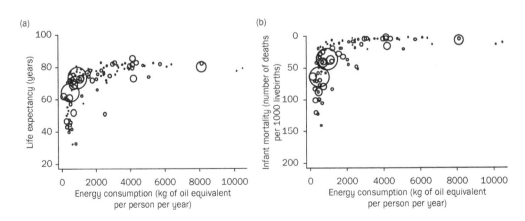

Figure 11.2 Energy consumption is positively associated with indicators of good health,
including (a) life expectancy and (b) infant mortality, although the marginal benefits decrease
with increasing consumption.

Source: Wilkinson et al. (2007).

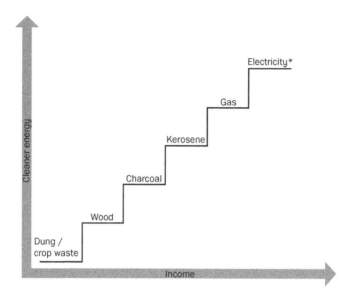

Figure 11.3 The energy ladder.

*Depending on the fuel used to generate it (e.g., electricty from coal will be less clean than other sources)

Source: Holdren and Smith (2000).

use a range of other study designs to investigate the distribution and determinants of energy-related ill health, from time-series and geographical studies common when exploring outdoor air pollution (see Chapter 7), to cohort and intervention studies. However, the analysis of accidents and natural experiments allows epidemiological investigations that would otherwise be unfeasible.

🖉 **Activity 11.2**

Read the following summaries of three examples where analyses of accidents, incidents and natural experiments have helped researchers understand energy–health associations, and evaluate their strengths and weaknesses in terms of study design, including their ability to provide robust evidence for the causation of health effects.

1 *The Chernobyl Nuclear Accident*: in 1986, an explosion at the Chernobyl nuclear power plant in the former USSR (now Ukraine) blew the roof off one of the reactors, spreading radioactive material over a wide area up to 2,000 km away. As a direct result of the explosion, there were two deaths and 134 reported cases of radiation sickness, 28 of whom died within three months. Marked increases in the incidence of

thyroid cancer have occurred in all areas of the Republic of Belarus and Ukraine, among all age categories, although the greatest increases have occurred among children. There was no excess leukaemia or other cancers found, contrary to what might have been expected from the experience of the nuclear bomb exposures.

2 *Ecuadorian oil fields*: billions of barrels of oil have been extracted from the Ecuadorian Amazon over the last three decades which has been accompanied by the release of enormous amounts of untreated waste and oil into the environment. Studies have found elevated cancer rates in residents living adjacent to oil fields when compared with expected population rates and also when compared to rates in counties without oil extraction activities (San Sebastián et al. 2001; Hurtig and San Sebastián 2002).

3 *Dublin coal ban*: on 1 September 1990, the Irish government banned coal sales in the city of Dublin, allowing researchers to compare air pollution and health impacts before and after the ban. The researchers found reductions in black smoke concentrations of 70 per cent and decreases in non-trauma death rates of 5.7 per cent. Respiratory and cardiovascular deaths decreased by 15.5 per cent and 10.4 per cent respectively (Clancy et al. 2002). However, subsequent analyses have suggested that broadly similar changes were observed elsewhere in Ireland.

Feedback

The examples above provided opportunities for epidemiological studies that might not have been available otherwise, for ethical or practical reasons. Exposing people to high levels of radiation or oil contamination is clearly ethically unacceptable, while implementing a pre-designed intervention study at a scale resembling the Dublin coal ban would be prohibitively expensive, as large sample sizes are often necessary to detect an association. Another advantage of studying these types of incident is that the impacts are seen in real populations rather than under artificial conditions characteristic of some study designs.

A key drawback of the evidence obtained from studying incidents and natural experiments is that their investigation is usually based on an interrupted time-series approach or similar, which looks for a before–after change, with or without comparison with a control area. In such circumstances, the potential for uncontrolled confounding is relatively high, and the evidence is correspondingly more difficult to interpret for cause-and-effect. When feasible, epidemiologists will often use other, more robust, study designs to try and confirm their findings such as randomized controlled trials and cohort studies.

In addition to the effects on the local resident population, occupational health is of concern in the energy sector because of the high risks associated with the extraction and processing of fossil fuels. Workers may also experience higher exposure to some hazards compared to members of the general population, for example to radiation at nuclear power facilities.

Health effects of specific energy types

Fossil fuels

The burning of fossil fuels, mainly for electricity generation, transport and home heating, is one of the major sources of outdoor air pollution (see Chapter 7) and has been the single greatest contributor to anthropogenic climate change (see Chapter 12). Natural gas is the cleanest in terms of both toxic pollutants and CO_2 emissions, while lignite and coal have the greatest emissions of air pollutants and CO_2 per TeraWatt hour of electricity production, with oil in between. The pollution generated depends on many factors including the amount of non-combustible material contained in the fuel; the type of burning technology used; any pollution control methods in place; and meteorological conditions.

Fossil fuel extraction, distribution and processing also carry substantial risks to health. Coal mining is associated with pneumoconiosis (black lung) and chronic obstructive pulmonary disease (COPD) (Donoghue 2004), while petroleum refining can release carcinogens such as benzene. Accidents in the fossil fuel sector contribute to injury and death, especially coal mining, which has been associated with substantial loss of life in recent years. In 2010 an explosion on the *Deepwater Horizon* oil rig in the Gulf of Mexico killed 11 workers and injured more than a dozen others. The subsequent oil spill released millions of barrels of oil into the Gulf. Although the long-term consequences of the spill will only be known in the future, hundreds of cases of illness were attributed to oil spill-related exposure, and there was also evidence for impacts on mental health in the local population along the Gulf Coast after the spill (Louisiana Office of Public Health 2010; National Commission on the BP *Deepwater Horizon* Oil Spill and Offshore Drilling 2011).

Fuel combustion for electricity generation is a key source of air pollution including sulphur dioxide and oxides of nitrogen, and the transport sector is a major emitter of carbon monoxide, oxides of nitrogen and volatile organic compounds (VOCs) (see Chapter 7). Both sectors contribute to particulate air pollution. Coal combustion also releases mercury, which if deposited in water can lead to exposure in humans through the consumption of contaminated fish. Lead (from leaded petrol) and mercury exposures cause neurological and developmental disorders. Household use of coal for heating or cooking exposes household members to indoor air pollution (now more commonly termed household air pollution) which is associated with cardio-respiratory diseases.

Indirect health impacts accompanying society's dependence on fossil fuels are also important. Motor vehicle crashes and reductions in physical activity from increased car dependence are discussed in more detail in Chapter 7. Fossil fuels have revolutionized agricultural production and food distribution and processing; increased food access benefits food-insecure populations, which is a considerable benefit to population health. However, cheap, energy-dense foods have also contributed to the increasing rates of obesity and non-communicable diseases seen in large parts of the world.

Nuclear power

The primary health concern from nuclear power is the release of radioactive material. Some radioactive isotopes have a long half-life, sometimes remaining in the environment for thousands of years. Exposure may take place via inhalation, external exposure from ground contamination or ingestion of foods from contaminated soil (Ahern et al. 2004). Exposure can lead to cancer and the potential for mutation, resulting in hereditary effects.

The fuel for nuclear power primarily comes from uranium mining, although other isotopic fuels are also generated in fast breeder reactors. Uranium mine workers have been shown to have an elevated risk of lung cancer in a number of studies (Ahern et al. 2004).

Fewer studies have been carried out on populations living near uranium mines, but soil samples taken from surrounding areas show higher levels of contamination than in control areas and residents may be exposed to low levels of radioactive contamination for many years.

There is also potential exposure to radionuclides from the waste materials from mining, processing and power generation. High-level waste material is destined for deep geological burial, although this is controversial because of public concerns about safety. A study of 90,000 US and European power station employees found that exposure to low-level doses of radiation over a long period of time increased their risk of developing leukaemia (Cardis et al. 1995).

Other concerns associated with nuclear power are its role in providing material for nuclear weapons, possible terrorism risks, escape of radionuclides into the environment and risk of reactor meltdown such as occurred at Chernobyl (see Activity 11.1) or the more recent incident at the Fukushima Daiichi power plant in Japan, in 2011. Although there were no immediate fatalities of the Fukushima incident, it led to high radiation exposures in some workers, and large-scale evacuation of the local area.

Renewable energy

Biomass (biofuels) Biomass refers to energy produced by burning organic matter such as wood, dung or agricultural waste. In many low-income countries biomass comprises the main source of household fuel, and is used for cooking and space heating. The United Nations Development Program estimates that 3 billion people rely on solid biomass fuels for cooking, as these materials are low cost and easily available. The health impact of air pollution produced from biomass burning and measures for control are discussed in more detail in Chapter 6.

Although still a small proportion of global energy supply, the use of solid biomass in high-income countries using modern technology, either in power plants or in the home, has increased in recent years due to fluctuations in the price of oil and concern about greenhouse gas emissions. (Biomass fuels are sometimes considered 'carbon-neutral' assuming that the same amount of emissions released from their combustion are later absorbed from the atmosphere during growth of new vegetation, although this does fully account for changes in land-use.)

Another recent development is the large-scale production of liquid biofuels for use in the transport sector. There are two main types of liquid biofuel, both of which are currently made primarily from food crops. Bioethanol is produced through a fermentation process that turns starches or sugars, mainly from maize or sugarcane, into ethanol. Biodiesel is produced from oil crops such as rapeseed, soya or oil palm.

The differences in vehicular air pollution between using biofuels and fossil fuels depends on the type of vehicle and other operating conditions, but it appears that burning liquid biofuels results in fewer particle (PM) emissions, but may increase emissions of ozone precursors.

Another key health concern of liquid biofuels relates to nutrition impacts from biofuel-induced food-price inflation that results from competition with the energy market for land and agricultural commodities. However, 'second-generation' biofuels, which can be produced from agricultural waste or dedicated non-food energy crops, are likely to become economically viable in the coming years and this could reduce pressure on food prices.

Hydroelectricity Hydroelectricity can only be produced where there is water and altitude – the electricity comes from harnessing the potential energy of water as it falls. Harnessing this energy requires building a dam to create a reservoir of water, which is then forced to flow through pipes that spin turbines. Many large-scale hydroelectric schemes provide both hydroelectric power and a clean water supply. Hydroelectricity is also a clean source of energy as it does not produce air pollutants. Nevertheless, the magnitude of infrastructure required, the changes such projects create in terms of land and water use, as well as any social disruption or dislocation that may occur, means that hydroelectric projects can contribute to ill health (see Table 11.1).

The construction of dams also raises questions about the 'ownership' of water sources, as rivers and watersheds often span multiple countries, meaning that restricting flows upstream can compromise water security for countries and populations downstream.

Table 11.1 Environmental and health impacts from hydroelectricity production

Environmental impact	Human health impact
Flooding from dam failure	Loss of life and injury
Changed environmental conditions for water- and vector-borne diseases	Increase in infection/transmission
Decreased natural fertilization of downstream agricultural land	Reduced crop planting/food supply
Loss of agricultural and other land	Reduced ability to grow food or graze animals
Changes in fish abundance and harvest	Changed fishing potential
Contamination of aquatic ecology and green house gas (GHG) emissions due to decay of flooded vegetation biomass	Reduced harvest, indirect effect on health through climate change
Occupational accidents during construction of dams and reservoirs	Death and injury
Dust and air pollution from construction and road building	Respiratory symptoms
Increased transport of building materials along roads (air pollution and accidents)	Respiratory symptoms, injury
Population displacement for dam construction and reservoir filling	Psychological and economic stress

Source: After Smith et al. (2013)

Other renewables Renewable energy harnesses energy forms that are non-depletable over the human timescale, and include wind and wave energy as well as solar energy. Biomass and hydroelectric energy, described above, are also considered renewable.

Although renewables still comprise only a small proportion of the world's energy supply, the sector is growing quickly. The cost of renewables is decreasing with improved technology, while the cost of fossil fuels is increasing due to the depletion of easily accessible reserves and the externalities associated with pollution and climate change (see Chapter 2 for an explanation of externalities).

In terms of health impact, renewables have a number of advantages over fossil fuels. As no combustion is required to produce the electricity except from biomas, renewables do not have an adverse impact on air quality; there is no air pollution or GHG emissions other than those embodied in the infrastructure. A further benefit of certain renewables is that they allow people to contribute to the provision of clean, sustainable energy at the individual level, without major infrastructure investments. For example, photovoltaic panels can be fitted to the roof of virtually any residence to provide solar power, and farmers and other landowners can erect wind turbines to provide wind power.

Indirect health impacts

In addition to the direct health impacts already discussed, dependence on fossil fuels has also been blamed for conflict within and between countries, and their contribution to climate change will contribute to future health burdens (see Chapter 12). Lastly, the energy industry strongly influences economic conditions, whether through income paid to governments, oil-price fluctuations or the behaviour of individual companies. In fact, it is difficult to identify health-related areas of life not influenced by energy policy, which has prompted epidemiologist Howard Frumkin to remark that 'Energy policy is health policy' (Frumkin 2011). For example, a substantial reduction in road deaths among children between 1975 and 1981 in New Zealand was not due to increases in road safety but because traffic levels had declined as a result of measures to limit car use in response to the oil price shocks of the 1970s (Roberts et al. 1992). Thus the observed decline in mortality was largely a result of reduced exposure to traffic as a result of current energy policy.

Evaluating energy policies

As we have seen, decisions about energy and energy policy have conse-quences reaching far beyond the energy sector. As a result, energy policies are usually designed with multiple objectives in mind, and decision-makers therefore have to weigh the merits of different policy options. Health scientists are sometimes asked to quantify the likely health impacts that may result from a given policy. Such an evaluation is known as a health impact assess-ment (HIA) (see Chapters 2 and 7). The type of decision that a given HIA is used to inform may range from evaluating specific pollution control measures or energy-efficiency interventions (see Table 11.2), to broad-scale decisions outlining strategies for energy security and sustainable development.

Concerns about the growing costs of fossil fuel combustion mean that there is increasing attention on decisions determining future methods of energy production. When evaluating the health impacts of different produc-tion alternatives, it is important to use a life cycle approach to assessment, which ensures that all stages in a fuel's life cycle are evaluated, from pros-pecting and extraction (or construction in the case of nuclear or renewables) through to end-use. Comparing only a single stage can provide misleading results because the stage in the life cycle where the main health impacts occur may vary across different options, resulting in underestimates of health burdens.

Figure 11.4 illustrates the life cycle of liquid biofuels, beginning with feed-stock production – growing the crops used for the biofuel – and finishing with its combustion in automobiles. From the perspective of air pollution, the diagram indicates that only assessing the end-use (combustion) stage would be a mistake; emissions also occur at all the other stages in the life cycle, from those emitted from on-farm machinery and during the refining process, to the trucks used to transport the feedstock and fuel. In Brazil, where bioethanol is made from sugarcane, sugarcane fields are often burned to facilitate harvest, and this has been linked to increases in hospital visits for respiratory complaints and hypertension in communities surrounding sugarcane fields (Arbex et al. 2006; Cançado et al. 2006).

Policies aimed at improving energy efficiency, which attempt to increase the amount of work provided per unit of energy, are another key strategy in

Table 11.2 Select pollution control and/or energy efficiency measures available in different energy sectors

Energy sector	Pollution control measures
Transport	Eliminating lead from petroleum Blending petroleum with liquid biofuels Use of ultra-light vehicle materials Hybrid-, electric- or hydrogen-powered vehicles Switching to active travel (walking/cycling)
Residential/buildings	Insulation Solar panels LED light bulbs Fuel switching
Electricity generation	Use of smokestacks in power stations Scrubbers Cogeneration Renewables

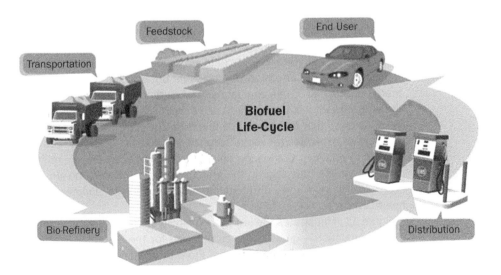

Figure 11.4 Illustration of the life cycle of liquid biofuel.

Source: Biofuels *Alternative Energy News* (2006–15).

achieving health- and sustainability-related objectives. Examples of energy efficiency policies range from insulating buildings and improving technologies (Table 11.2), to implementing labelling standards on household appliances to allow informed consumer choices. From a health perspective, there are few drawbacks to improving energy efficiency in principle, although HIAs are still an important tool to help choose between competing policies and for identifying the most appropriate means of implementation.

An important feature of energy efficiency policies is that even if they do succeed in reducing the energy demanded for a given task, this does not necessarily reduce the *total* energy demand – lower costs may stimulate increased demand. Nevertheless, most countries have reduced their energy intensity (energy use per $ of GDP) since 1990, and the World Energy Council estimates that productivity improvements from 1990–2006 resulted in both savings of 4.4 gigatonnes of oil equivalents globally and avoided the release of 10 gigatonnes of CO_2 (World Energy Council 2008).

Health impact assessment of energy policies and co-benefits

The previous discussion concentrated on assessing health impacts when public health is an explicit consideration of a potential energy policy. However, HIA can also be used to quantify any co-benefits (or dis-benefits) that may accrue from policies designed or implemented for other purposes. Estimating co-benefits is a way to further support policies that may be beneficial across multiple spheres or can determine if a policy is likely to cause an unexpected adverse health impact.

In the energy sector, and with regard to climate change in particular, it appears that strategies to reduce GHG emissions often have favourable co-benefits to human health. For example, a case study in Delhi, India, showed that prioritizing active transport and low-emission vehicles positively impacts on physical activity, air pollution and road safety, while case studies from the UK and Brazil have demonstrated that reducing consumption of livestock products, which are GHG intensive, can lower the risk of ischaemic heart disease (Friel et al. 2009; Woodcock et al. 2009). Similar findings have been demonstrated with regards to electricity generation and household energy use (Markandya et al. 2009; Wilkinson et al. 2009) (Activity 11.3).

Activity 11.3

In order to meet climate change mitigation targets, richer countries will have to reduce their GHG emissions substantially over the coming decades. In the UK, residential buildings account for an estimated 26 per cent of total emissions, over half of which come from space heating.

A number of strategies exist to improve household energy efficiency thereby reducing GHG emissions. Four key strategies include: increased insulation; improved ventilation control; fuel switching (to electricity); and discouraging occupants from keeping homes above a temperature threshold (18°C) in winter.

Think about these four mitigation strategies and describe potential health co-benefits or dis-benefits that may occur from their implementation.

Feedback

Potential health co-benefits include the following.

*   *Insulation:* changes to indoor temperature through reduced heat loss which directly impacts temperature-related mortality (deaths increase at high and low temperatures) and indirectly affects mould growth.
*   *Ventilation:* affects indoor air quality (including particles, radon, etc.), temperature and mould growth.
*   *Fuel switching:* removal of combustion-related indoor air pollutants.
*   *Occupant behaviour:* the impacts on health of keeping indoor temperatures to a recommended threshold are not entirely clear but could influence temperature-related mortality (Wilkinson et al. 2001).

A health impact study quantified the effect of simultaneously implementing all four of the above strategies at a level that would enable substantial reductions in GHG emissions (Wilkinson et al. 2009). The researchers estimated that this combined strategy would result in 850 fewer disability-adjusted life years (DALYs) per million population over a one-year period when compared to a scenario where UK housing and population health did not change. The researchers used the same pathways to health described above.

Energy and sustainable development

Energy and sustainability are inextricably linked, in terms of both the sustainability of human populations and the broader environment. We have already discussed the importance of renewable energy and energy efficiency in mitigating dangerous climate change and reducing other forms of pollution. Reducing energy demand is a third strategy, and while this is feasible to some extent in richer populations, it must be balanced against the need for more energy in populations facing fuel poverty. Accordingly, energy-related sustainable development is a central tenet of Goal 7 of the Sustainable Development Goals (SDGs), to 'ensure access to affordable, reliable, sustainable and modern energy for all' (UN 2015).

The rapid increase in global energy production and consumption has been associated with an increase in environmental degradation, including impacts beyond air pollution and climate change. As with health impacts, environmental degradation can occur at any stage in the life cycle of an energy source, and pressures on the environment come in many forms – some of these are given in Table 11.3.

The scale of global energy use means that energy-related environmental degradation has contributed to substantial biodiversity loss and a reduction in ecosystem services (see Chapter 13).

Table 11.3 Some key environmental concerns attributed to different energy sources

Energy source	Environmental concerns
Petroleum	Deforestation from extraction Oil spills from extraction and distribution Air pollution (including GHGs) from combustion
Coal	Air pollution (including GHGs) from combustion Production of large amounts of waste such as fly-ash
Natural gas	Water usage and water pollution from fracking* Air pollution (including GHGs) from combustion
Hydroelectric	Land-use change (e.g. conversion of rivers to reservoirs) Loss of natural water and nutrient flows
Nuclear	Release of radiation Radioactive waste
Solid biomass	Deforestation Air pollution from combustion
Liquid biofuels	Direct and indirect land-use change including deforestation Air pollution from combustion
Solar photovoltaic	Changes to land cover
Wind power	Changes to land cover Potentially dangerous to birds/bats in flight

* See Activity 11.4 for explanation of this term

 Activity 11.4

New drilling techniques have only recently enabled energy companies to profitably extract natural gas trapped in rock crevices situated thousands of feet underground. The process, called hydraulic fracturing, or 'fracking', entails drilling a well shaft into the rock and pumping in water and chemicals to open cracks that will release the gas. An average well uses millions of gallons of water and tens of thousands of gallons of chemicals.

After injection, the water is returned to the surface for treatment or re-use.

Whether to allow fracking has become a hotly debated topic in many parts of the world, with particularly vocal protests in parts of the USA, Australia and a dry region of South Africa called the Karoo, among others.

Note some potential advantages and disadvantages of this technique. Consider impacts on human health and the environment.

Feedback

Many of the issues around fracking are still under investigation, but the main concerns include:

- *Contamination of ground and surface water* with fracking chemicals or methane released from the rock. Although fracking normally occurs far below aquifers used for drinking water, there is concern that pollutants can migrate upwards through cracks in the rock, or more likely through poorly sealed or previously decommissioned wells. Moreover, the injected fluid is brought back to the surface after use, where it is often stored in open pits which risk overflow during heavy rains. Although many of the chemicals are unknown and protected as trade secrets, some are known or suspected human carcinogens.
- *Depletion of local water supplies*: the quantity of water necessary is large and in arid areas, such as South Africa's Karoo, residents worry about the loss of water entitlements for household or agricultural uses. Reduced water supply can affect aquatic ecosystems.
- *Air (and GHG) emissions* from methane leaks and machinery. VOCs present in gas reservoirs can also enter the fluid and be released into the air during evaporation from surface pits.
- *Occupational accidents* associated with drilling or potential chemical exposure.

Potential advantages include:

- *Increased access to energy through increased supply and/or lower prices*: about 1.5 billion people in developing countries still lack access to electricity including populations in South Africa and other countries considering fracking.
- *Burning natural gas releases fewer emissions than its alternatives*: for example, South Africa relies heavily on coal which is a dirtier energy source than natural gas.
- *Job creation.*
- *Reduced dependence* on oil-exporting countries.

Summary

In this chapter you have been introduced to key concepts in the energy sector. Energy consumption has increased rapidly over the last 200 years, with most of the energy provided by fossil fuels. But as the continuing use of fossil fuels has started to undermine many of the benefits they helped to achieve, there is a trend towards renewable energy sources. Renewable energy sources provide opportunities to improve health and reduce pressures on the environment, but still comprise only a fraction of total energy consumption. Due to the wide-reaching impacts of decisions taken in the energy sector, it is important to balance health considerations with those in other sectors, particularly the environmental, social and economic impacts.

References

Ahern, M. et al. (2004) Exposure and health impacts of electric power generation, transmission and distribution, in B. Menne and A. Markandya (eds) *Energy, Sustainable Development and Health*. Geneva: WHO.

Alternative Energy News (2006–15) http://www.alternative-energy-news.info/technology/biofuels/, accessed 6 December 2015.

Arbex, M. et al. (2010) Impact of outdoor biomass air pollution on hypertension hospital admissions, *Journal of Epidemiology and Community Health*, 64(7): 573–9.

Cançado, J. et al. (2006) The impact of sugar cane burning emissions on the respiratory system of children and the elderly, *Environmental Health Perspectives*, 114(5): 725–9.

Cardis E. et al. (1995) Effects of low doses and low dose rates of external ionizing radiation: cancer mortality among nuclear industry workers in three countries, *Radiation Research*, 142(2): 117–32.

Clancy, L. et al. (2002) Effect of air-pollution control on death rates in Dublin, Ireland: an intervention study, *Lancet*, 360(9341): 1210–14.

Donoghue, A. (2004) Occupational health hazards in mining: an overview, *Occupational Medicine*, 54(5): 283–9.

Friel, S. et al. (2009) Public health benefits of strategies to reduce greenhouse-gas emissions: food and agriculture, *Lancet*, 374(9706): 2016–25.

Frumkin, H. (2011) Stop Washington state coal-energy production, *Seattle Times*.

Holdren, J.P. and Smith, K. (2000) Energy, the environment, and health, in J. Goldemberg (ed.) *The World Energy Assessment: energy and the challenge of sustainability*, pp. 61–110. New York: UN Development Programme.

Hurtig, A.K. and San Sebastián, M. (2002) Geographical differences in cancer incidence in the Amazon basin of Ecuador in relation to residence near oil fields, *International Journal of Epidemiology*, 31(5): 1021–7.

IEA (2012) Statistics and balances, http://www.iea.org/stats/graphsearch.asp, accessed 17 August 2012.

Louisiana Office of Public Health (2010) Louisiana DHH releases oil spill-related exposure information. Baton Rouge, LA: Louisiana OPH.

Markandya, A. et al. (2009) Public health benefits of strategies to reduce greenhouse-gas emissions: low-carbon electricity generation, *Lancet*, 374: 2006–15.

National Commission on the BP *Deepwater Horizon* Oil Spill and Offshore Drilling (2011) *Deep Water: the Gulf oil disaster and the future of offshore drilling*. New Orleans, LA: National Commission on the BP *Deepwater Horizon*.

Roberts, I., Marshall, R. and Norton R. (1992) Child pedestrian mortality and traffic volume in New Zealand, *British Medical Journal*, 305: 283.

San Sebastián, M. et al. (2001) Exposures and cancer incidence near oil fields in the Amazon basin of Ecuador, *Occupational and Environmental Medicine*, 58(8): 517–22.

Smith, K.R., Frumkin, H., Balakrishnan, K. et al. (2013). Energy and human health, *Annual Review of Public Health*, 34: 159–88.

UN (2015) Sustainable Development Knowledge Platform, https://sustainabledevelopment.un.org/?menu=1300, accessed 12 January 2016.

Wilkinson, P. et al. (2001) *Cold Comfort: the social and environmental determinants of excess winter deaths in England, 1986–1996*. UK: Policy Press.

Wilkinson, P. et al. (2007) A global perspective on energy: health effects and injustices, *Lancet*, 370(9591): 965–78.

Wilkinson, P. et al. (2009) Public health benefits of strategies to reduce greenhouse-gas emissions: household energy, *Lancet*, 374(9705): 1917–29.

Woodcock, J. et al. (2009) Public health benefits of strategies to reduce greenhouse-gas emissions: urban land transport, *Lancet*, 374(9705): 1930–43.

World Energy Council (2008) *Energy Efficiency Policies around the World: review and evaluation*. London: World Energy Council.

Global climate change and stratospheric ozone depletion

12

Sari Kovats

Overview

Human activity is changing the climate system. In this chapter, we discuss anthropogenic climate change caused by emissions of greenhouse gases (GHGs) and stratospheric ozone depletion caused by production of synthetic chemicals. Climate change is likely to have important but complex implications for public health through impacts on extreme weather, food security and infectious disease. An international environmental agreement has successfully reduced emissions of ozone-depleting substances. Policies to address climate change (adaptation and mitigation) are being implemented but emissions of GHGs are still increasing. We explore the implications of climate policies for human health, and highlight the potential benefits to public health.

Learning objectives

By the end of this chapter you will be able to:

- describe the causes of global climate change and its effects on human health
- describe the causes of stratospheric ozone depletion and its effects on human health
- understand some of the main approaches to estimating the impact that large-scale environmental changes may have on health in the future
- understand the two policy approaches to addressing climate effects on health (adaptation and mitigation)
- appreciate health inequalities associated with future impacts of climate change

Key terms

Adaptation: Adjustment in natural or human systems in response to actual or expected climate change, in order to reduce harm or exploit beneficial opportunities.

Climate change: Refers to any change in climate over time, whether due to natural variability or as a result of human activity. Anthropogenic climate change is a change in climate caused by human activity.

Mitigation: An intervention to reduce the anthropogenic climate change or other environmental hazard. For example, strategies to reduce GHG emissions and enhance GHG sinks.

Scenario: A plausible and often simplified description of how the future may develop, based on a coherent and internally consistent set of assumptions about driving forces and key relationships.

Stratospheric ozone depletion: Depletion of the ozone layer in the stratosphere, caused by the action of synthetic chemicals such as chlorofluorocarbons (CFCs), and leading to increased UVR reaching the Earth's surface.

Ultraviolet radiation (UVR): Electromagnetic radiation with a wavelength shorter than that of visible light, but longer than X-rays, that is, in the range 10 nm to 380 nm.

Introduction

This chapter addresses two global environmental problems that affect human health: anthropogenic climate change and stratospheric ozone depletion. Both problems involve the climate system but in different ways, consequently the causes and the effects on health are very different, as are the policy solutions. For each problem, we give a brief explanation of how each occurs, discuss the health implications, and then consider responses in the context of public health policies.

Climate change: background

Climate change is caused by the build-up of heat-trapping (greenhouse) gases in the lower atmosphere (see Figure 12.1). It is a global problem because emissions of GHGs mix in the lower atmosphere and affect the global climate system, irrespective of where they have been emitted. For more information on the causes of climate change and climate science see the reports of the Intergovernmental Panel on Climate Change (IPCC 2014). The greenhouse gases, some of which are produced by human activity, include carbon dioxide (CO_2), methane (CH_4), nitrous oxide (N_2O), water vapour (H_2O), ozone (O_3) and CFCs.

Box 12.1: What drives climate change?

Figure 12.1 demonstrates how the radiative balance between incoming solar shortwave radiation (SWR) and outgoing longwave radiation (LWR) is influenced by global climate 'drivers'. Natural fluctuations in solar output (solar cycles) can cause changes in the energy balance (through fluctuations in the amount of incoming SWR). Human activity changes the emissions of gases and aerosols, which are involved in atmospheric chemical reactions, resulting in modified ozone and aerosol amounts. Anthropogenic changes in GHGs (e.g. CO_2, CH_4, N_2O, O_3, CFCs) and large aerosols (>2.5 μm in size) modify the amount of outgoing LWR by absorbing outgoing LWR and re-emitting less energy at a lower temperature.

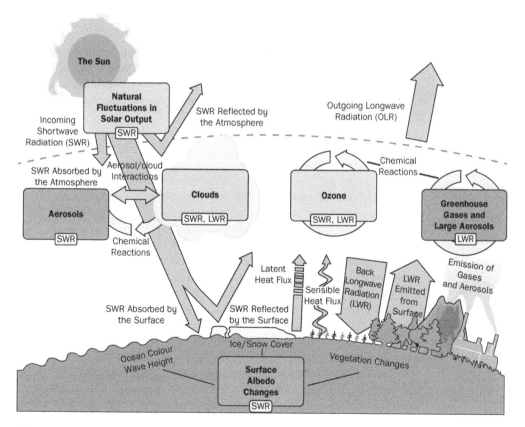

Figure 12.1 The main drivers of climate change.

Source: Cubasch et al. (2013, Figure 1.01).

As we consider climate change, it is important to distinguish between the different concepts of 'climate' and 'weather'. Weather is the temperature or rainfall and state of the atmosphere on a given day in a specific place. Climate is the average weather in a given location, typically defined over a 30-year period. Climate *change* is defined as a statistically significant variation in either the mean state of the climate or in its variability, persisting for an extended period (typically decades or longer) (IPCC 2014). Climate change may be due to either natural internal processes or external forces (as shown in Figure 12.1). External forces include persistent human-induced changes in the composition of the atmosphere (due to GHG emissions, or deforestation that reduces the capacity of the land to act as a carbon sink). The international environmental agreement on climate change (the United Nations Framework Convention on Climate Change or UNFCCC) defines climate change as: 'changes in climate caused by human activities' (UN 1992). For the purposes of this chapter, we will use this definition and discuss only anthropogenic climate change.

Estimating future climates

Climate science uses computer models to project future possible climates, based on assumptions about future GHG emissions. Climate scientists estimate the following changes this century, based on the latest scientific assessment by the Intergovernmental Panel on Climate Change (IPCC 2013):

- Increase of global mean surface temperatures for 2081–2100 relative to 1986–2005 is to likely be in the range 1.1°C to 4.8°C.
- Global mean sea level will continue to rise during the twenty-first century and the rate of sea level rise will very likely exceed that observed between 1971 and 2010 due to increased ocean warming and increased loss of mass from glaciers and ice sheets.
- It is virtually certain that there will be more frequent hot and fewer cold temperature extremes over most land areas on daily and seasonal timescales as global mean temperatures increase. It is very likely that heatwaves will occur with a higher frequency and duration. Occasional cold winter extremes will continue to occur.

Figure 12.2 shows the range of uncertainty around the future projections of average global temperature. The main source of uncertainty is the amount of future GHG emissions (the range illustrated by representative concentration pathways (RCPs) scenarios in the figure). It is important to note that significant differences are projected between regions, with rates of warming highest in the polar regions, and northern Canada and Europe. The future impact of climate change on local and regional weather patterns will vary depending on location and time. It is very likely to lead to warmer summers, milder winters, and more hot days and fewer cold days. In addition,

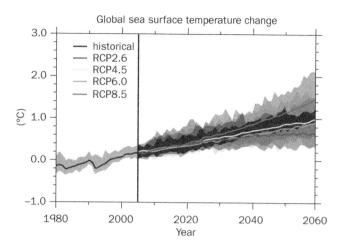

Figure 12.2 Projected changes in annual averaged, globally averaged, surface ocean temperature based on selected climate models, under four twenty-first century scenarios of future GHG emissions (RCP 2.6, RCP 4.5, RCP 6.0 and RCP 8.5) (shading illustrates the 90 per cent range of projections against the 1986–2005 average).

Source: Kirtmann et al. (2013).

there may be an increase in the frequency and intensity of some types of extreme weather events (droughts, floods, windstorms).

Health effects of climate change

Many health outcomes are affected by weather patterns and extreme weather events. Table 12.1 summarizes what we currently know about the effects of temperature and rainfall factors (weather) on human health, based on observational epidemiological studies.

Climate change is a very complex environmental hazard that will affect health through many different pathways (see Figure 12.3). It will affect a variety of traditional environmental hazards, including heat and cold (temperature extremes), and air quality, as well as the transmission of vector-borne and water-borne diseases (see Chapter 5 on water and sanitation) (Smith et al. 2014).

Climate change is a regional and long-term phenomenon (lasting decades or longer). When considering future impacts on health, it is important not to simply extrapolate what we know now about the sensitivity of populations to climate and weather. For example, the response of a population to high temperatures will change over time due to acclimatization and improvements to housing and the built environment. For a comprehensive assessment of climate change impacts on health, one must also consider the future health status of the population of interest.

Table 12.1 Current evidence regarding the impact of temperature and rainfall on health

Health outcomes	Known effects of weather and climate variability
Acute mortality risks	Daily death rates from cardio-respiratory causes increase with high and low temperatures Heat-related morbidity and mortality (hyperthermia, heat injuries) due to heatwaves Morbidity and mortality (hypothermia) due to cold
Air pollution-related mortality and morbidity	Weather affects local air pollutant concentrations; temperature and rainfall affect atmospheric chemistry and dispersion of pollutants Weather and climate affect distribution, seasonality and production of aeroallergens
Mortality, injuries, infectious diseases, mental health	Natural disasters (floods, windstorms) cause deaths (e.g. by drowning) and injuries, and long-term psychological morbidity, and also affect health through damage to infrastructure (e.g. damage to housing, sanitation systems, hospitals, etc.)
Vector-borne diseases (e.g. malaria, dengue)	Higher temperatures reduce the development time of pathogens in vectors and increase potential transmission to humans Vector species require specific climate conditions (temperature, humidity) to be sufficiently abundant to maintain transmission; high temperatures may alter the distribution of vector species
Water/food-borne diseases	Survival of important bacterial pathogens is increased with higher temperatures Extreme rainfall can affect the transport of disease organisms into the water supply; heavy rainfall associated with outbreaks of water-borne disease; low rainfall associated with diarrhoeal disease when there is a lack of water for hygiene Increases in drought conditions may affect water availability and water quality (chemical and microbiological load) due to extreme low flows
Food security	Drought and flood events can lead to crop losses leading to local food shortages which can affect calorie intake and micro-nutrient deficiency

Source: Modified from Kovats and McMichael (2010)

 Activity 12.1

Consider your country in the last 10 years. What major climate-related events (disasters) have occurred? What were the main health impacts? How is this vulnerability likely to change in the next 10 years? What about the next 50 years?

Feedback

Some communities are better able to cope with major weather disasters than others. You may have described the following events and impacts.

- *Type of event*: floods are the most common natural disaster, and can be caused by heavy rainfall or a storm surge in coastal areas. High temperatures cause heatwaves which can be accompanied by wild-fires and drought events.
- *Impacts of the event on health*: mortality, injuries, infectious diseases, temporary population displacement in shelters and associated effects.
- *Destruction of critical infrastructure*: damage to hospitals, energy supply and roads may also have implications for health.

You may have considered whether vulnerability (in terms of the impact of a given event) may increase or decrease over the next 10 years, based on what has happened in the past 10 years (the continuation of the current trend). Imagining impacts 50 years hence is much more difficult. It is possible that current trends will continue but it is also possible that some unexpected changes may occur. This is why scenarios are used in order to help describe the future impacts of climate change.

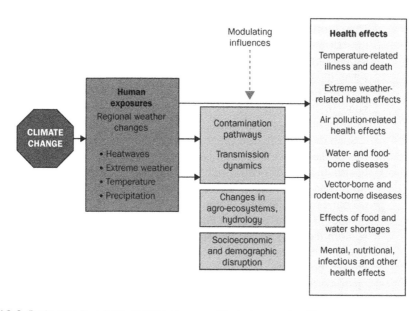

Figure 12.3 Pathways by which climate change affects human health.
Source: Kirtmann et al. (2013).

Policy responses to climate change

Adaptation to climate change

Climates have changed over millennia. The Earth has experienced ice ages and periods of warming in the past. The problem we are facing now is the rate of change in the climate, which may be a faster rate than some populations can adapt to. There may also be limits to how much climate change populations are able to adapt to. Adaptation is defined as activities, processes or adjustment in natural or human systems in response to actual or expected climate change, in order to reduce harm, improve health and wellbeing, or exploit beneficial opportunities (Campbell-Lendrum et al. 2007). For example, raising coastal flood defences to prevent flooding from sea-level rise is an adaptation. Public health activities that improve resilience to extreme weather events and climate variability are also considered as adaptation (Hess et al. 2012), and are illustrated in relation to heatwaves and malaria in the following sections.

The impact of higher temperatures on human health: heatwaves

Over the past 20 years, the countries in Europe and North America have experienced an increase in the frequency of very hot days, consistent with the observed trend in warming (IPCC 2012, 2013). There is much research on the association between environmental temperatures and daily mortality. The evidence from most countries suggests that mortality risk increases at high and low extremes of temperature. Europe has experienced several major heatwaves in recent years: the major heatwave in 2003 caused approximately 35,000 deaths across western Europe (Robine et al. 2008) and a major heatwave and air pollution episode in 2010 was associated with 11,000 excess deaths in Moscow (Shaposhnikov et al. 2014).

Such recent heatwave events provide opportunities to identify what effective public health measures can be implemented to reduce or prevent the health impacts of heatwaves. In 2003, France experienced a 20-day heatwave (see also Chapter 6). During the heatwave, the daily death rate was 60 per cent higher than normal, with 14,802 extra deaths compared to the number of deaths expected during this time period. The health surveillance system did not register the actual number of deaths occurring in a timely way and consequently did not act as an alerting mechanism to the major impact on health from the heatwave. An effective health surveillance system, together with the appropriate use of meteorological (weather) forecasts, provide advance warning of high temperatures, and are part of any effective plan for managing a heatwave (see Chapter 10 on disasters). Table 12.2 describes the core elements of a national heat health plan in more detail.

Table 12.2 Core elements of a heat health plan

1	Agreement on a lead body (responses to heatwave need to consider multiple agencies)
2	Accurate and timely alert systems (heat-health warning systems trigger warnings, determine the threshold for action and communicate the risks)
3	A heat-related health information plan (about what is communicated, to whom and when)
4	A reduction in indoor heat exposure (medium- and short-term strategies) (advice on how to keep indoor temperatures low during heat episodes)
5	Particular care for vulnerable population groups
6	Preparedness of the health and social care system (staff training and planning, appropriate health care and the physical environment)
7	Long-term urban planning (to address building design and energy and transport policies that will ultimately reduce heat exposure)
8	Real-time surveillance and evaluation

Source: Matthies et al. (2008).

The impact of higher temperatures on human health: malaria

Many important infectious diseases that are transmitted by insect or tick vectors are sensitive to climate factors (Table 12.1). Malaria is caused by a parasite (*Plasmodium* spp.) that is transmitted from person to person by the female *Anopheles* mosquito. There are approximately 1 million deaths each year as a result of malaria, mostly in children (Lozano et al. 2012). In recent decades, the incidence and distribution of malaria has declined due to intervention measures (such as vector control measures, new treatments and the use of insecticide treated bednets). However, in some areas there has been a resurgence of malaria due to drug and insecticide resistance.

The use of geographical information system (GIS) technology to map environmental data (such as satellite data) means that disease risk maps can be created in order to target control measures. The distribution of malaria has been mapped in Africa using parasite surveys, which have then been validated (Hay et al. 2009). At the continental scale, climate is a determinant of malaria distribution and transmission intensity. However, at the local level, other factors become more important, such as the presence of lakes and other sources of mosquito breeding sites. The northern distribution of malaria in Africa is limited by the Sahel, which is too dry for mosquitoes to transmit the disease. The southern distribution is limited by control measures, which reduce transmission, particularly in South Africa (Moonasar et al. 2012).

Malaria transmission is also affected by temperature and rainfall factors on a seasonal basis in many areas, with a peak associated with the arrival of the rainy season. Outbreaks of malaria have also been associated with heavy rainfall (extreme weather) events. For example, in 1998, a drought was followed by heavy rainfall and flooding in arid Wajir County, Kenya, and the failure to implement vector control programmes immediately led to a very large epidemic of malaria (Maes et al. 2014).

Climate change may affect future malaria incidence in the following ways.

- Increasing its *distribution*. Where epidemic malaria is currently limited by temperature, it may become present in new areas. As temperatures increase, mosquitoes can survive in areas which previously were too cold, and malaria transmission can take place in those areas.
- Decreasing the *distribution* where it becomes too dry for mosquitoes to be sufficiently abundant for transmission.
- Increasing or decreasing the months of transmission.
- Increasing the risk of local outbreaks in areas where disease is eradicated but vectors are still present, for example, in southern Europe or the USA.

These assessments are confirmed by observations of long-term trends in climate and effects on malaria transmission. For example, an increase in the altitude of malaria distribution has been observed in the highlands of Colombia and Ethiopia that can be attributed to higher temperatures (Siraj et al. 2014). In the next section, we will look at the methods used to quantify the potential effects of climate change on population health in the future.

Assessing future risks to health from climate change

In this section, we illustrate the difficulties in projecting the future impact of climate change on human health outcomes, using malaria as an example.

Figure 12.4 shows a malaria distribution in Africa under current and future climate scenarios (Tanser et al. 2003). Climate scenarios are plausible and consistent descriptions of the future global climate. The figure shows that the distribution of malaria may expand in the East African highlands. The distribution may also be reduced at its northern limits due to projected decreases in rainfall. The modelling study does not take into account future actions to control malaria.

There are several sources of uncertainty in assessing future impacts. The main ones are:

- Unknown future GHG emissions, and therefore the future climate changes (increased temperature and rainfall changes) that populations will experience. Figure 12.4 shows three different climate futures, based on three different scenarios of GHG emissions to get a range of future possible climate change.
- Natural climate variability. Year to year variations can be large, and this is why 30-year averages are used in the assessment.

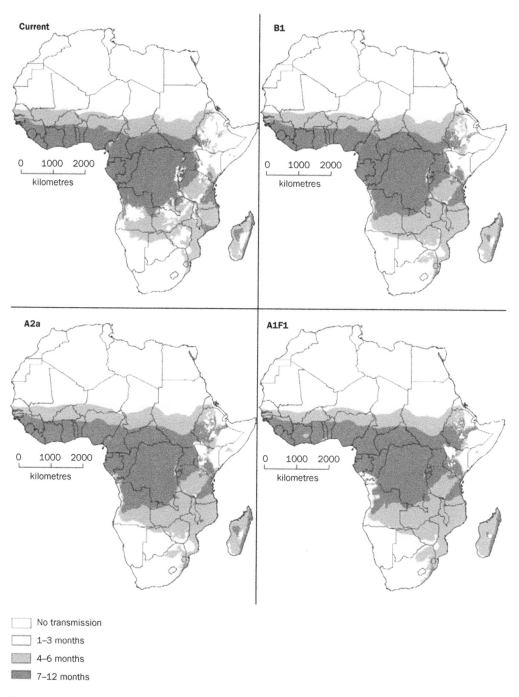

No transmission

1–3 months

4–6 months

7–12 months

Figure 12.4 Estimated number of months suitable for *Plasmodium falciparum* transmission by 2100 using three emission scenarios (low: B1, medium: A2a, high: A1F1).

Source: Adapted from Tanser et al. (2003).

- Different responses between different global climate models. In Figure 12.4, only one climate model is used (HadCM3) and it would be better to use a range of climate models to capture a larger range of possible climate futures.
- Poorly resolved regional and local climate changes (e.g. the climate scenarios may not represent accurately the future climate change in local areas or in highland areas).
- Possibility of abrupt, non-linear changes in the climate system (not included in scenarios).
- Changes in important non-climate factors for malaria (e.g. land use change) are not represented in the model.
- Changes in disease control measures are not represented in the model.

The existence of uncertainties does not imply the absence of knowledge; we understand some aspects of future climate change better than others. For example, there is more confidence in the models of future increases in CO_2 concentrations and temperature than in modelled increases in changes in rainfall.

Climate scenarios and impact assessment

Climate scenarios are generally derived from the output of global or regional climate models. National climate scenarios are specifically constructed for national impact assessments. The first generation of climate scenarios described changes in average conditions, but the latest scenarios now include estimates of changes in the magnitude and occurrence of extreme weather events, as well as probabilistic projections.

As nearly all aspects of our natural, physical and social environments will change in the future, it is important that changes are reflected in the scenarios used in climate impact studies. Population growth and economic growth (in GDP/capita) are also routinely included in climate impact studies. A limitation of these studies is that they must make assumptions about how future populations will respond to exposure to high temperatures, including the rate of acclimatization and adaptation.

Box 12.2: Advantages and disadvantages of using climate change scenarios

Advantages:

- *articulate key considerations and assumptions*:
  o scenarios can help to imagine a range of possible futures if we follow a key set of assumptions and considerations

- *blend quantitative and qualitative knowledge*:
  - ○ scenarios are powerful frameworks for using both data and model-produced output in combination with qualitative knowledge elements
- *identify constraints and dilemmas*:
  - ○ exploring the future often yields indications for constraints in future developments and dilemmas for strategic choices to be made
- *expand our thinking beyond the conventional paradigm*:
  - ○ exploring future possibilities that go beyond our conventional thinking may result in surprising and innovative insights.

Disadvantages:

- *lack of diversity*:
  - ○ scenarios are often developed from a narrow, disciplinary-based perspective, resulting in a limited set of standard economic, technological and environmental assumptions
- *extrapolations of current trends*:
  - ○ many scenarios have a 'business-as-usual' character, assuming that current conditions will continue for decades
- *inconsistent*:
  - ○ sets of assumptions made for different sectors, regions or issues are often not consistent with each other
- *not transparent*:
  - ○ key assumptions and underlying implicit judgements and preferences are not made explicit
  - ○ it may not be clear which factors or processes are exogenous or endogenous, and to what extent societal processes are autonomous or influenced by concrete policies.

Stratospheric ozone depletion and ultraviolet radiation (UVR): background

The synthetic chemicals CFCs were developed in the 1930s. At the time, they were rigorously tested for toxicity and teratogencity. CFCs were inert and non-toxic, and therefore widely used as refrigerants, anaesthetics, solvents, propellants and in polystyrene manufacture. However, in 1974, Molina and Rowland argued that when CFCs were exposed to UVR at low temperatures they would release free chlorine radicals which catalyse the breakdown of ozone in the atmosphere (Farman 2005).

The stratosphere is the region of atmosphere extending from about 10 km to 50 km. It contains a layer of ozone (O_3) formed by the action of UVR on oxygen. The ozone layer acts as a screen which absorbs a lot of the UVR from the sun, and prevents it from reaching Earth's surface. In a cold atmosphere, the free radicals from the CFCs react with the ozone layer. This has led to a thinning of the ozone layer, particularly over the poles and in springtime. The 'ozone hole' refers to the thinning of the ozone layer above Antarctica from September to December each year.

Policy actions to address stratospheric ozone depletion and UVR

In 1985, the Vienna Convention for the Protection of the Ozone Layer was the first international environmental agreement (IEA) to be signed before full scientific data were available on the effects. This use of the precautionary principle (Chapter 2) was based on projections of future ozone depletion, as well as the robust knowledge that UVR is biologically damaging to all animal and plant species (Farman 2005). The discovery of rapid and severe seasonal destruction of ozone over Antarctica was first reported in 1985, and the Montreal Protocol, phasing out CFCs, was ratified in 1987.

The monitoring of emissions, concentrations and the thickness of the ozone layer is important to ensure compliance with the international environmental agreement and its amendments. Unlike GHGs, CFCs were from relatively few sources and easier to regulate, because effective and cheap alternatives were available.

The effects of stratospheric ozone depletion on health

The health effects of ozone depletion are both direct and indirect (Norval et al. 2011). Direct effects include skin cancer, eye damage and damage to the immune system. Indirect effects from the impact of increasing UVR include damage to terrestrial and aquatic systems, which themselves generate further consequences for the environment and human health. UVR can be classified into three types depending on the wavelength: UVA, UVB, and UVC.

Quantitative risk estimates are available for some of the UVB-associated effects – for example, skin cancer – based on epidemiological studies that have quantified risks in a variety of populations (Armstrong and Kricker 2001). UVR also causes damage to the eye, including chronic eye conditions such as cataract, squamous cell carcinoma, ocular melanoma and a variety of corneal/conjunctival effects.

Suppression of local (at the site of UV exposure) and systemic (at a distant, unexposed site) immune responses to a variety of antigens has been demonstrated in both humans and animals exposed to UVB. There is reasonably good evidence that such immunosuppression plays a role in human carcinogenesis; however, the implications of such immunosuppression for human infectious diseases are still unknown (Norval et al. 2011).

The main health concern regarding increased UVR for human populations is the impact on skin cancer, with evidence to suggest that increases in risk are tied to early exposures (before about age 15), particularly those leading to severe sunburns (Norval et al. 2011).

✎ Activity 12.2

Quantitative risk estimates have been developed for cataract, melanoma and all skin cancers combined. Figure 12.5 describes projections of future impacts of ozone depletion on skin cancer under a range of policies (amendments and protocols relating to the international environmental agreement the Vienna Convention for the Protection of the Ozone Layer, also known as the Montreal Protocol). What are the health benefits of regulating CFC emissions?

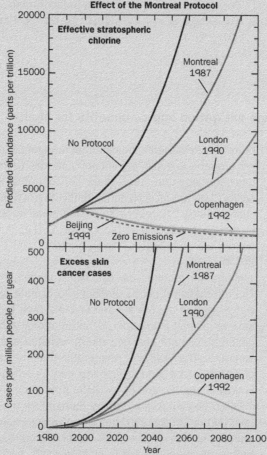

Figure 12.5 Future excess skin cancer attributable to stratospheric ozone depletion.

Source: WMO (2003).

Feedback

- These estimates indicate that, under the Copenhagen amendment, skin cancer incidence is projected to peak just after mid-century at an additional incidence of under 100 cases per million people per year.
- Estimated additional burden under the no-action scenario is compared to burdens under international action (as described by the Montreal Protocol and its amendments) represented in the figure.
- The impacts are felt in the populations at different times. Note also that there is a time lag from emissions to ozone depletion and from UV exposures in individuals to the development of cancer (about 20 years).

Climate change mitigation and co-benefits for health

Current assessments indicate that substantial reductions in GHG emissions are required to avoid 'significant' changes to the climate system. The IPCC has estimated that atmospheric concentration levels of about 450 ppm CO_2 eq by 2100 are broadly consistent with a likely chance to keep temperature change below 2°C relative to pre-industrial levels. This can only be achieved by substantial cuts in anthropogenic GHG emissions by mid-century through large-scale changes in energy systems and potentially in land use (IPCC 2014).

Mitigation requires constructive engagement at the international level. The international policy response to climate change is the UNFCCC which was signed at the Rio summit in 1992 (see Table 14.1 in Chapter 14), and sets an overall framework for international efforts to tackle the challenge posed by climate change, and is revisited each year in the global climate summits. The UNFCCC recognizes that the climate system is a shared global resource whose stability can be affected by industrial and other emissions of CO_2 and other GHGs from each country. The UNFCCC meeting in 2015 has led to the Paris Agreement for the reduction of climate change (and carbon emissions), the text of which represented a consensus of the representatives of the 196 parties (countries) attending the meeting. Before the meeting, 146 countries (high, middle and low income) publicly presented draft national climate contributions (called 'Intended Nationally Determined Contributions', INDCs) that specified local actions to reduce carbon emissions.

Emissions reduction can be achieved in a number of ways such as changing the technologies used, making use of energy-efficient processes and moving away from carbon-based fuels to increased use of wind, solar and other renewable sources (see Chapter 11). It is also important to preserve carbon sinks such as forests (carbon sequestration is an 'ecosystem service', see Chapter 13).

Climate change and health inequalities

Climate change will not have an equal effect across the environment and different populations of the globe. The ability of a country or a region to cope with climate change depends on its wealth, technology and infrastructure. Low- and middle-income countries, historically, did not have the industry, transportation or intensive agricultural practices that are the causes of climate change, and so have made little contribution to the total (historic) GHG emissions. However, low-income countries may have limited capacity to protect themselves against the adverse consequences of climate change and may be particularly vulnerable to the effects.

The effects of climate change on human health are complex and will depend upon the capacity of the population to address environmental problems. There are large differences in the projected impacts between high- and low-income countries.

- For example, a rise in sea level is likely to affect densely populated populations in low-lying deltas, such as in Bangladesh, which are more difficult to protect, whereas in other countries such as the Netherlands, where most of the population is settled on land below sea level, the people are protected by flood defences that are built to withstand a 1 in 1,000 year event.
- The impacts of climate change on cereal crop yields are projected to be largely negative at low latitudes, where crops are near their temperature tolerance limit. In contrast, climate change may increase crop yields in high latitudes, at least in the first half of this century.

The international equity issues of climate change are very important (Tóth 1999). These issues are formally recognized within the UNFCCC, because high-income countries have agreed to help low-income countries to adapt.

 Activity 12.3

Actions to address climate change are a challenge for environmental and health equity. What questions arise from the impact of and response to climate change?

Feedback

- *Intergenerational equity.* What is the responsibility of current generations to future generations? Is it fair that the current generation experiences the benefits of a fossil-fuel intensive world, while future generations may suffer from climate change?
- *International equity.* Historically, from past emissions, climate change has been caused mainly by the high-income industrialized countries. However, it is the poorer countries which are likely to be more affected by adverse impacts. What responsibilities do the 'polluters' have for the countries most affected by climate change? For example, should high-income countries provide financial support to low-income countries to help them adapt to climate change?
- Are low-income countries entitled to industrialize and to the benefits from energy-intensive economies that high-income countries enjoy, and can they therefore defer their actions to mitigate climate change? Is it possible to have clean energy and economic development?

Summary

Climate change and stratospheric ozone depletion are both large-scale and long-term phenomena that have direct and indirect health consequences. International environment agreements have been established to address climate change and stratospheric ozone depletion. However, while international cooperation has led to a successful ban on the emissions of ozone-depleting substances, there has been less agreement regarding actions to reduce GHG emissions. The issues of sustainable development and equity are also important considerations for policies to respond to global environmental changes.

References

Armstrong, B.K. and Kricker, A. (2001) The epidemiology of UV induced skin cancer, *Journal of Photochemistry and Photobiology B: Biology*, 63(1–3): 8–18.

Campbell-Lendrum, D., Corvalán, C. and Neira, M. (2007) Global climate change: implications for international public health policy, *WHO Bulletin*, 85(3): 235–7.

Cubasch, U., Wuebbles, D., Chen, D. et al. (2013) Introduction, in T.F. Stocker et al. (eds) *Climate Change 2013: the physical science basis*. Contribution of Working Group I to the Fifth Assessment Report of the Intergovernmental Panel on Climate Change. Cambridge: Cambridge University Press.

Farman, J. (2005) Halocarbons, the ozone layer and the precautionary principle, in *Late Lessons from Early Warning*. Copenhagen: EEA.

Fouillet, A., Rey, G., Wagner, V. et al. (2008) Has the impact of heat waves on mortality changed in France since the European heat wave of summer 2003? A study of the 2006 heat wave, *International Journal of Epidemiology*, 37(2): 309–17.

Haines, A. et al. (2009) Public health benefits of strategies to reduce greenhouse-gas emissions: overview and implications for policy makers, *Lancet*, 374: 2104–14.

Hay, S.I., Guerra, C.A., Gething, P.W. et al. (2009) A world malaria map: *Plasmodium falciparum* endemicity in 2007, *PLoS Medicine*, 6(3): e1000048.

Hess, J., McDowell, J.Z. and Luber, G. (2012) Integrating climate change adaptation into public health practice: using adaptive management to increase adaptive capacity and build resilience, *Environmental Health Perspectives*, 120(2): 171–9.

IPCC (2012) *Managing the Risks of Extreme Events and Disasters to Advance Climate Change Adaptation. A Special Report of Working Groups I and II of the Intergovernmental Panel on Climate Change.* Cambridge: Cambridge University Press.

IPCC (2013) Summary for policymakers, in T.F. Stocker et al. (eds) *Climate Change 2013: the physical science basis.* Contribution of Working Group I to the Fifth Assessment Report of the Intergovernmental Panel on Climate Change. Cambridge: Cambridge University Press.

IPCC (2014) Summary for policymakers, in O. Edenhofer et al. (eds) *Climate Change 2014: mitigation of climate change.* Contribution of Working Group III to the Fifth Assessment Report of the Intergovernmental Panel on Climate Change. Cambridge: Cambridge University Press.

Kirtman, B., Power, J.A., Adedoyin, G.J. et al. (2013) Near-term climate change: projections and predictability, in T.F. Stocker et al. (eds) *Climate Change 2013: the physical science basis.* Contribution of Working Group I to the Fifth Assessment Report of the Intergovernmental Panel on Climate Change. Cambridge: Cambridge University Press.

Kovats, R.S. and McMichael, A.J. (2010) Climate change, in J. Ayres, R. Harrison, G. Nichols and R. Maynard (eds) *Environmental Medicine*, pp. 510–20. London: HodderArnold.

Lozano, R. et al. (2010) Global and regional mortality from 235 causes of death for 20 age groups in 1990 and 2010: a systematic analysis for the Global Burden of Disease Study, *Lancet*, 380(9859): 2095–128.

Maes, P., Harries, A.D., Van den Bergh, R. et al. (2014) Can timely vector control interventions triggered by atypical environmental conditions prevent malaria epidemics? A case-study from Wajir County, Kenya, *PLoS One*, 9(4): e92386.

Moonasar, D. et al. (2012) Malaria control in South Africa 2000–2010: beyond MDG6, *Malaria Journal*, 11: 294, doi:10.1186/1475-2875-11-294.

Norval, M., Lucas, R.M., Cullen, A.P. et al. (2011) The human health effects of ozone depletion and interactions with climate change, *Photochemical and Photobiological Sciences*, 10: 199–225.

Patz, J.A. et al. (2000) The potential health impacts of climate variability and change for the United States: executive summary of the report of the health sector of the U.S. National Assessment, *Environmental Health Perspectives*, 108(4): 367–76.

Robine, J.M., Cheung, S.L.K., Le Roy, S. et al. (2008) Death toll exceeded 70000 in Europe during the summer of 2003. *Comptes Rendus Biologies*, 331: 171–8.

Shaposhnikov, D., Revich, B., Bellander, T. et al. (2014) Mortality related to air pollution with the Moscow heat wave and wildfire of 2010, *Epidemiology*, 25(3): 359–64.

Siraj, A.S., Santos-Vega, M., Bouma, M.J., Yadeta, D. and Ruiz Carrascal, D.W. (2014) Altitudinal changes in malaria incidence in highlands of Ethiopia and Colombia, *Science*, 343(6175): 1154–8.

Smith, K.R., Woodward, A., Campbell-Lendrum, D. et al. (2014) Human health: impacts, adaptation, and co-benefits, in C.B. Field et al. (eds) *Climate Change 2014: impacts, adaptation, and vulnerability. Part A: global and sectoral aspects*, pp. 709–754. Contribution of Working Group II to the Fifth Assessment Report of the Intergovernmental Panel on Climate Change. Cambridge: Cambridge University Press.

Tanser, F.C., Sharp, B. and le Sueur, D. (2003) Potential effect of climate change on malaria transmission in Africa, *Lancet*, 362(9398): 1792–8.

Tóth, F. (ed.) (1999) *Fair Weather: Equity concerns in climate change.* London: EarthScan.

UN (1992) The United Nations Framework Convention on Climate Change, FCCC/INFORMAL/84. New York: United Nations, http://unfccc.int/key_documents/the_convention/items/2853.php.

UNEP/WMO (2010) *Assessment of the Scientific Panel*. Nairobi: UNEP.

WMO (World Meteorological Organization) (2003) *Scientific Assessment of Ozone Depletion: 2002*, Global Ozone Research and Monitoring Project, WMO Report 47, p. 498. Geneva: WMO.

Ecosystem services and public health

13

Carolyn Stephens and Sari Kovats

Overview

This chapter describes the interactions between the natural environment and human health. The ecosystem services framework can be used to describe the many different benefits that the natural environment provides for human health and wellbeing. There are three main ecosystem services: provisioning services (e.g. providing food and shelter); regulating services (such as the water and carbon cycles); and cultural services which, for example, include the mental health benefits of contact with nature. Human activities are changing the natural environment, and can lead to loss of ecosystem services with implications for biodiversity and human health.

Learning objectives

By the end of this chapter you will be able to:

- describe the linkages between human activities, the natural environment and human health
- critically evaluate the concept of ecosystem services
- assess the implications of biodiversity loss and deforestation for human health

Key terms

Biodiversity: Variability among living organisms, including the variability within and between species and within and between ecosystems.

Ecosystem: The interactive system formed from all living organisms and their abiotic (physical and chemical) environment within a given area.

Ecosystem services: The benefits that people obtain from the natural environment, including provisioning services such as water and food.

Green spaces: Areas of grass, trees or other vegetation set apart for recreational or aesthetic purposes or for the control of hazards (e.g. natural flood management) in an otherwise urban environment.

Ecosystem services: an introduction

Ecosystem services are indispensable to the wellbeing of all people, everywhere in the world. They include provisioning, regulating, and cultural services that directly affect people, and supporting services needed to maintain the other services. From the availability of adequate food and water, to disease regulation of vectors, pests, and pathogens, human health and wellbeing depends on these services and conditions from the natural environment. Biodiversity underlies all ecosystem services.

(WHO 2012)

The ecosystem services framework was first developed for the United Nations' Millennium Ecosystem Assessment (MEA). The objective of the MEA was to assess the current state of ecosystems and the large-scale trends that are causing environmental degradation and biodiversity loss (see Chapter 3). Further, the MEA aimed to assess the scientific basis for action needed to protect ecosystems and enhance the sustainable use of those systems. The ecosystem framework was used to describe (and quantify) the value of a robust and healthy ecosystem to human health and wellbeing. It describes the many different benefits that the natural environment provides to human populations.

The natural environment is a general term to describe ecosystems – the interactive systems formed from all living organisms and their abiotic (physical and chemical) environment within a given area. Ecosystems cover a hierarchy of spatial scales and can comprise the entire globe, biomes at the continental scale or small, well-circumscribed systems such as a small pond. Ecosystems include tropical rainforests (such as the Amazon rainforest), mangrove forests and also urban environments.

Human populations benefit greatly from the natural environment. However, these benefits are not always obvious and therefore an attempt has been made to make the pathways (or services) more explicit. These ecosystem services can be organized into three main types:

- *provisioning services*: ecosystems provide food (crop production, fisheries), energy (biofuels) and materials for shelter (wood) and clothing;
- *regulating services*: ecosystems are essential for ensuring clean water and clean air, and regulating the carbon cycle and the nitrogen cycle;
- *cultural services*: natural landscapes and urban green spaces provide educational, spiritual, aesthetic and recreational services.

The loss of ecosystem services (through environmental degradation and destruction) can also increase the risk of disasters. It is therefore important to maintain the ecosystem service of 'hazard control' to protect populations from natural disasters (this is discussed in more detail in Chapter 10). Mangroves are an example of an ecosystem that provides protection from storm damage by buffering the impacts of coastal storms.

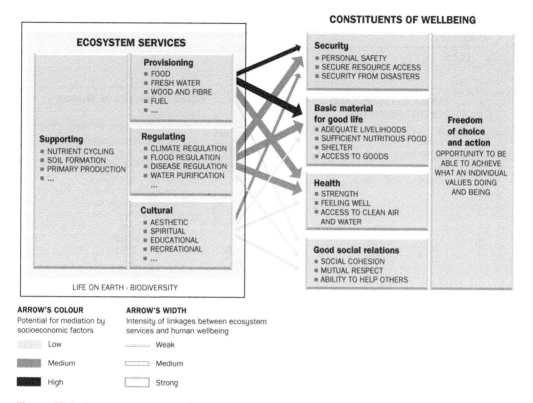

Figure 13.1 Ecosystem services for health and wellbeing.

Source: WHO (2005).

Figure 13.1 depicts the ecosystem services framework and the links to human health and wellbeing for each of the three types of ecosystem service. The strength of these links is illustrated by the width of the arrow. The diagram also shows that most of these relationships are mediated or affected by social and economic factors. For example, clean (safe) fresh water is vital for human health, but access to safe water for an individual is strongly mediated by household income and urban planning, which are in turn determined by socioeconomic factors (see Chapter 5 on water and sanitation).

The natural environment is also affected by human activity. Figure 13.2 shows how these ecosystems services interact at different scales and over time. It also describes some of the drivers of change (these were introduced in Chapter 3). Social, demographic, natural and political processes can profoundly affect our ecosystem services, both directly and indirectly. For example, urbanization and population growth may increase demands for fresh water, leading to over-extraction of water in rivers that harms fish and other aquatic species. It is estimated that between 5 and 25 per cent of current global water consumption and up to 35 per cent of global irrigation withdrawals exceed sustainable levels (WHO 2012). Freshwater depletion has repercussions in terms of desertification, loss of wetlands, damaging forest cover and increasing the risk of wildfire.

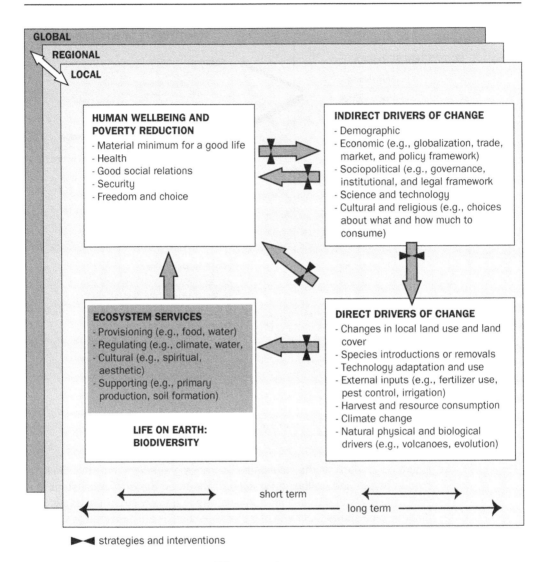

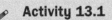 strategies and interventions

Figure 13.2 Ecosystem services at different scales.
Source: WHO (2012).

✐ **Activity 13.1**

Consider the following extract and Figure 13.1. Summarize the constituents of wellbeing linked to food, and the ways in which human activity can affect the availability of food through changing the natural environment.

Human interventions are altering the capacity of ecosystems to provide their goods (e.g. freshwater, food, pharmaceutical products, etc.) and services (e.g. purification of air, water, soil, sequestration of pollutants, etc.). Ecosystem disruption can impact on health in a variety of ways and through complex pathways. The types of health effects experienced are determined by the degree to which local populations depend on ecosystem services, and factors such as poverty which affect vulnerability to changes in elements like access to food and water.

Feedback

Productive terrestrial and marine ecosystems, both wild and managed, are the source of our food through agriculture and fisheries/aquaculture, respectively. Food production is an essential ecosystem service and prerequisite for health and life. Human activities can affect the natural environment (leading to a loss of ecosystem services) in a number of ways:

- land use change – loss of agricultural land through urbanization or desertification which affects crop production;
- deforestation may affect access to wild foods;
- over-fishing can lead to dramatic drops in stocks of fish due to over-exploitation of the marine ecosystem;
- climate change is likely to have an impact on food production in the future;
- freshwater depletion can lead to reduced crop production – if fresh water becomes contaminated with chemicals or saltwater, this may have a consequent negative impact by causing contamination of the food chain.

The MEA was a scientific assessment of the state of the natural environment at the global scale. It was used to provide scientific evidence to support international agreements such as the Convention on Biodiversity (see below and Chapter 14, Table 14.1). Some countries have also undertaken a scientific assessment of ecosystem services at the national scale. The UK published a National Ecosystem Assessment which included consideration of the value of ecosystems to human health (Pretty et al. 2012). In high-income countries, there has been an increased interest in the public health benefits of contact with nature, including blue space (lakes, oceans), forests and urban green spaces (Hartig et al. 2014).

The importance of access to green space within an urban environment was discussed in Chapter 9. Access to green space is an important component of the spatial determinants of health in urban areas (Grant et al. 2009). The nature of the built environment (including urban green space) affects the determinants of health in urban settings through, for example, the ability of people to walk and cycle (active travel), to have access to healthy food and to be part of a supportive community (Hartig et al. 2014).

 Activity 13.2

Read the extract below from the UK National Ecosystem Assessment (Pretty et al. 2012) and answer the questions that follow.

The UK national ecosystem assessment concluded that ecosystems provide three generic health benefits:

i) Direct positive effects on mental health and physical health
ii) Indirect positive effects
   a) Facilitating nature-based activity and social engagement (by providing locations for contact with nature, physical activity and social engagement), all of which positively influence health.
   b) Providing a catalyst for behavioural change in terms of encouraging the adoption of healthier lifestyles (improving life pathways, activity behaviour and the consumption of wild foods).
iii) Reducing the threats and incidence of pollution and disease vectors via a variety of purification and control functions such as local climate regulation, noise reduction and absorbing of air pollutants.

1 What are the key health issues that have been identified for the UK population and how do these differ from health issues that are linked to ecosystem services in a low-income country?
2 What type of scientific evidence do you think was used in the assessment?

Feedback

1 The key health issues that the assessment identified for the UK population include the direct benefits to non-communicable diseases in the UK population, particularly increases in physical activity and improvements in mental health from green spaces in urban areas. It is likely that an assessment in a low-income country may be more focused on infectious diseases, and issues of water availability and water quality.
2 Several types of evidence would be used to support the findings of the assessment, these would include:
   • epidemiological studies that detect and quantify the association between green spaces and mental health or physical activity or related health outcomes;

- ecological studies of ecosystems and vector abundance;
- qualitative research on the effect of the natural environment (forests, green spaces) on people's wellbeing and social integration.

Biodiversity and human health

Biodiversity refers to the multiplicity of species, plants and animals in a biological community and the ecological niches that they occupy. Many ecologists argue that diversity in animal and plant species leads to greater stability of the ecosystem (Ives and Carpenter 2007). More complicated systems may have greater adaptability in the face of environmental changes, because ecological niche occupants may overlap to some extent and allow substitutions if one or more are lost. There is currently some debate whether biodiversity should be included as an ecosystem service or as part of the natural capital from which services flow. Ecologists do agree, however, that biodiversity losses within an ecosystem have adverse effects on service provision (Mouillot et al. 2013).

It is difficult to make direct links between aspects of biodiversity and human health because effects operate at different scales and intensities of relationship, and the scientific evidence base is limited (Lovell et al. 2014). Humans have been cultivating and collecting plants and animals for their own purposes for thousands of years: to treat disease (quinine for example), act as pesticides (neem for example), or provide shelter or clothing uses (sisal, cotton, hemp, or grass).

Nearly every area of medicine relies on natural products to develop clinical treatments, but dependence on natural products has been particularly heavy for antibiotics and anticancer drugs (Bernstein 2014). Once a plant has been identified as useful to humans, there is a danger that it will become extinct. The cinchona tree was harvested almost to the point of extinction before the Dutch made a very successful plantation in Java that supplied 90 per cent of all quinine until the 1940s. Yacón is a tuber of the Andes, almost forgotten outside of Latin America until very recently, and now being investigated for its properties for treating diabetes, for colon and intestinal health and for cancer (Genta and Cabera 2009).

Biodiversity allows plant and animal species to adapt and develop into new or changed ecosystems. For thousands of years, humans have intervened in this natural biodiversity to increase food production or quality – for example, careful breeding of wild strains of grain has meant that agricultural practices can develop and spread into new areas. Wheat, maize and rice provide half of the world's food, and new ways have been found to substantially increase yields. For example, monoculture grain production can lead to large-scale yields but can also mean that the crops are vulnerable to disease. In some areas this has meant vast areas planted in single varieties; while this has meant increases in yield and ease of harvesting, it has also meant the potential loss of some cultivars as well as the opportunity for pest or disease outbreaks to devastate whole areas. To ensure food security, we need to preserve the genetic diversity of plants and animals. There are now seed banks throughout the world, collecting as many different cultivars as possible and storing them.

Human activity has been a key determinant of biodiversity loss either directly or indirectly. Biodiversity loss is considered to be one of the planetary boundaries that has been exceeded (see Chapter 3). Individual species have become extinct through habitat loss, or reduction in the species that they depend on for food, or through human hunting for food or pleasure, or chemical contamination of land and/or water habitats. Entire ecosystems or vast areas of larger ecosystems may be changed or lost through urbanization and agricultural clearance, with particular habitats of individual species with limited habitat ranges destroyed. Climate change may also affect habitat characteristics, leading to widespread changes in the local ecosystem, and subsequent biodiversity loss.

Critical understanding of ecosystem services

There is a need to improve understanding of the importance of biodiversity and ecosystem services for human health and wellbeing. It has been argued that this need to quantify or value the benefits from nature is especially urgent in fragile and vulnerable ecosystems, such as forests, where communities depend directly on the resources of their environment (UNEP-WCMC 2011). Some argue that only a human-centred, or anthropocentric, view of the ecosystem will enable decision-makers to prioritize ecosystem conservation and enhance sustainable ecosystems. However, it can be argued that biodiversity has a value independent of its relationship to human wellbeing (Rudd 2011).

Much conservation policy is focused on protecting species and ecosystems for their intrinsic value. Species and ecosystems have 'intrinsic value' – a value 'in and for itself' (Callicott 1988) and there is an ethical obligation to protect biodiversity. Some scientists now advocate controversial conservation strategies such as triage (prioritization of species that provide unique or necessary functions to ecosystems) (Bottrill et al. 2008; Parr et al. 2009).

Deforestation and human health

The MEA estimated that 'In the last three centuries, global forest area has been reduced by approximately 40%, with three quarters of this loss occurring during the last two centuries. Forests have completely disappeared in 25 countries, and another 29 countries have lost more than 90% of their forests' (Shvidenko et al. 2005) (see Figure 13.3).

In contrast to loss of biodiversity (where species extinctions cannot be reversed), there are significant opportunities to regenerate forests. Thus, while some regions are experiencing rapid deforestation, others are regenerating forests after centuries of destruction. The Sustainable Development Goal (SDG) 15 is to sustainably manage forests, with a target to halt deforestation, restore degraded forests and substantially increase afforestation and reforestation globally by 2020. In the past 10 years the proportion of land covered by forest has decreased less rapidly at a global level, and quite marked reductions have occurred in South East Asia and Latin America. Restoring forests does not mean that the same ecosystems can be regenerated: forests provide some of the world's most biodiverse ecosystems and when they are destroyed it is not just the trees that need to be regenerated.

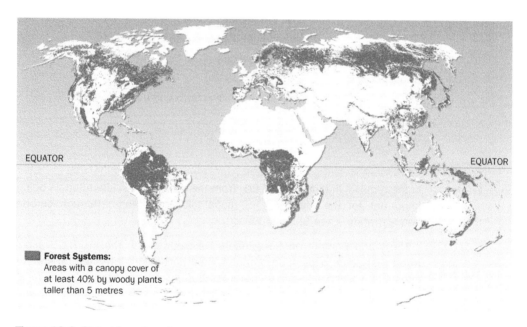

EQUATOR   EQUATOR

Forest Systems:
Areas with a canopy cover of
at least 40% by woody plants
taller than 5 metres

Figure 13.3 Global forest systems.
Source: Millennium Ecosystem Assessment (2007).

Deforestation has many consequences (see Table 13.1). Deforestation in tropical areas has immediate local effects – there is increased soil erosion (due to decreases in soil stability from roots and resulting decreased protection against the effect of wind and rain) and resultant sedimentation of rivers with loss of plants and animals. Tropical forests have some of the richest ecosystems on Earth, and while they can regenerate after clearing, the same biodiversity cannot be restored. Forests also have a critical role

Table 13.1 Consequences of tropical deforestation

Effects	Consequences
Local effects	Soil erosion by gullies and slopewash
	Small slope failures
	Accelerated loss of sediment
	Less infiltration and increased run-off
	Loss of soil fertility
Regional effects	Large slope failures via mass movement and debris flows
	Increased flooding in rivers
	Alteration of river characteristics
	Coastal sediment problems
	Loss of regional flora and fauna
	Alteration of lifestyle of local inhabitants
	Climatic changes
Global effects	Loss of biodiversity
	Loss of carbon sink and contribution to global climate change

Source: Gupta and Asher (1998)

in the removal and storage of CO_2 from the atmosphere, identified as being important for the mitigation of global climate change (through carbon sequestration – see Chapter 12).

The World Summit on Sustainable Development in Rio in 2012 recognized that some population groups will be particularly affected by loss of ecosystem functions such as deforestation: 'indigenous peoples and local communities are often the most directly dependent on biodiversity and ecosystems and thus are often the most immediately affected by their loss and degradation' (UN 2012).

There is also good evidence that community protected forests can have benefits locally as well as internationally (Shvidenko et al. 2005; Stolton and Dudley 2010). For example, Amazonia is one of Earth's most important biodiverse, tropical, moist forest ecosystems. As the Amazonian forest reaches the Andes it becomes a contiguous and equally vital ecosystem: the Yungas or Cloud Forest (Fundacion Proyungas 2007). These two sister forests are among the most biodiverse ecosystems of the world. For millennia, the Amazonia/Yungas has been protected by over 1,000 different indigenous peoples (Montenegro and Stephens 2006). In turn, Amazonia/ Yungas has provided health and wellbeing for indigenous peoples via food, medicines, home and culture (Stephens et al. 2003). These forests also provide the world with some of its most important ecosystem services in terms of forest and food resources, current and potential new medicines, rainfall regulation and a global carbon sink. Deforestation, resource extraction and climate change threaten all parts of the Amazonia/Yungas ecosystem. Indigenous communities, among the most marginalized peoples in Latin America (Hall and Patrinos 2005), are experiencing increasing threats to their territories and their health and wellbeing (Montenegro and Stephens 2006).

The destruction of biodiverse ecosystems is from a range of causes including deforestation, mining, resource extraction and 'biopiracy', generated by economic demand. High-income countries are currently particularly responsible for the resource extraction that impacts negatively on biodiversity and on the wellbeing of local communities (Witzig and Ascencios 1999). In terms of protection of these ecosystems, national and regional parks, reserves and conservation areas are very important, and local communities have a vital role to play in protection of the ecosystem in and around them. There is evidence that recognized 'indigenous territories' are better protected, in terms of biodiversity and environmental damage, than other conservation areas (Dunning et al. 2010; Ramos and Junqueira 2010).

Recognizing their vital role in ecosystem understanding and protection, indigenous peoples and local communities now play an important part in global policy processes, including the UN Convention on Biological Diversity (UNCBD) and the UNFCCC (Chapter 14). In 2011, the International Union for the Conservation of Nature (IUCN) met with indigenous representatives and conservation organizations to discuss conservation priorities in the context of indigenous rights, and to advance their implementation. These resolutions, along with the Durban Action Plan and the Programme of Work on Protected Areas of the UNCBD, were called a 'new conservation paradigm' (IUCN 2011).

Progress toward sustainable development and continued human wellbeing relies on the ability to maintain ecosystems and biodiversity. The demands on the ecosystem for the provision of water and food are growing, but human activity has degraded many ecosystems. Good management can reverse some damage and prevent more from occurring. The UNCBD is the international environmental agreement established to protect global biodiversity (see Chapter 14). It was designed to provide an international framework to halt biodiversity loss and the sustainable use and equitable sharing of the benefits. To achieve the targets agreed there needed to be monitoring and an understanding of the causal relationships between human activities and environmental change, along with the availability of options to prevent the loss of biodiversity. The MEA was established to improve the knowledge base, to understand the complicated relationship between ecosystems and human wellbeing and devise options for appropriate interventions. In 2012, under the UNCBD, countries agreed a new strategic plan for 2012–20 with specific targets (Aichi Biodiversity

Targets) and more participation of communities directly affected by eco-system damage.

Summary

This chapter has examined the concept of ecosystem services for describing the interactions between the natural environment and human health, and critically evaluated the role of this concept in ecosystem protection. While it is not presently possible to estimate with certainty the full effects of global environmental changes on health, the loss of biodiversity has already had an impact on the world's ecosystems. Indigenous communities have a vital role in conserving biodiversity and our forest ecosystems.

References

Bernstein, A. (2014) Biological diversity and human health, *Annual Review of Public Health*, 35: 153–67.

Grant, M., Barton, H., Coghill, N. and Bird, C. (2009) *Evidence Review on the Spatial Determinants of Health in Urban Settings*. Bonn: WHO European Centre for Environment and Health.

Bottrill, M.C. et al. (2008) Is conservation triage just smart decision making?, *Trends in Ecology and Evolution*, 23(12): 649–54.

Callicot, J. (1988) *On the Intrinsic Value of Nonhuman Species. The Preservation of Species: the value of biological diversity*. Princeton, NJ: Princeton University Press.

Dunning, E. et al. (2010) *The role of protected areas in mitigating climate change and conserving biodiversity. Everything is connected: climate and biodiversity in a fragile world*. London: DEFRA, http://sd.defra.gov.uk/2010/11/everything-is-connected-climate-and-biodiversity-in-a-fragile-world/.

Fundacion Proyungas (2007) *Bitácora de las Yungas: Bosques Nublados*. Tucuman: Fundacion de las Yungas.

Genta, S. et al. (2009) Yacon syrup: beneficial effects on obesity and insulin resistance in humans, *Clinical Nutrition*, 28(2): 182–7.

Gupta, A. and Asher, M. (1998) *Environment and the Developing World: principles, policies and management*. Chichester: John Wiley & Sons Ltd.

Hall, G. and Patrinos, H.A. (2005) *Indigenous Peoples, Poverty and Human Development in Latin America: 1994-2004*. Washington, DC: World Bank.

Hartig, T., Mitchell, R., de Vries, S. and Frumkin, H. (2014) Nature and health, *Annual Review of Public Health*, 35: 207–28.

IUCN (2011) IUCN to review and advance implementation of the 'new conservation paradigm' focusing on rights of indigenous peoples, http://www.iucn.org/about/union/commissions/ceesp/ceesp_news/?7399/IUCN-to-review-and-advance-implementation-of-the-new-conservation-paradigm, accessed 29 November 2011.

Ives, A.R. and Carpenter, S.R. (2007) Stability and diversity of ecosystem, *Science*, 317(5834): 58–62.

Lovell, R., Wheeler, B.W., Higgins, S.L., Irvine, K.N. and Depledge, M.H. (2014) A systematic review of the health and well-being benefits of biodiverse environments, *Journal of Toxicology and Environmental Health B: Critical Reviews*, 17(1): 1–20.

Millennium Ecosystem Assessment (2007) MA Synthesis Report Figures zip, http://www.millenniumassessment.org/en/GraphicResources.aspx, accessed 26 January 2017.

Montenegro, R.A. and Stephens, C. (2006) Indigenous health in Latin America and the Caribbean, *Lancet*, 367(9525): 1859–69.

Mouillot, D., Bellwood, D.R., Baraloto, C. et al. (2013) Rare species support vulnerable functions in high-diversity ecosystem, *PLoS Biology*, 11(5): e1001569, doi: 10.1371/journal.pbio.1001569.

Parr, M.J. et al. (2009) Why we should aim for zero extinction, *Trends in Ecology and Evolution*, 24(4): 181; author reply 183–4.

Pretty, J., Barton, J., Colbeck, I. et al. (2012) Health values from ecosystems, in *UK National Ecosystem Assessment*. Cambridge: UNEP-WCMC.

Ramos, A. and Junqueira, R. (2010) *The Contribution of Indigenous People to Forest Conservation and Recovery. Everything is Connected: climate and biodiversity in a fragile world*. London: DEFRA, http://sd.defra.gov.uk/2010/11/everything-is-connected-climate-and-biodiversity-in-a-fragile-world/.

Rudd, M.A. (2011) Scientists' opinions on the global status and management of biological diversity, *Conservation Biology*, 25: 1165–75.

Shvidenko, A. et al. (2005) *Forest and Woodland Systems. Ecosystems and Human Well-being: Current State and Trends: findings of the Condition and Trends Working Group* (R. Hassan, R. Scholes and N. Ash). Washington, DC: Island Press.

Stephens, C. et al. (2003) *Utz' Wach'il: health and well-being among indigenous peoples*. London: Health Unlimited and the London School of Hygiene & Tropical Medicine.

Stolton, S. and Dudley, N. (2010) *Arguments for Protection Vital Sites*. Oxford: World Wide Fund for Nature/Equilibrium Research.

UNEP-WCMC (2011) *Health and Wellbeing of Communities Directly Dependent on Ecosystem Goods and Services: an indicator for the Convention on Biological Diversity*. Cambridge: UNEP-World Conservation Monitoring Centre.

WHO (2005) *Ecosystems and Human Well-being: health synthesis*. Geneva: WHO.

WHO (2012) *Our Planet, Our Health, Our Future. Human Health and the Rio Conventions: biological diversity, climate change and desertification*. Geneva: WHO.

Witzig, R. and Ascencios, M. (1999) The road to indigenous extinction: case study of resource exportation, disease importation, and human rights violations against the Urarina in the Peruvian Amazon, *Health and Human Rights*, 4(1): 60–81.

SECTION 3

Policy

Action at global and local levels

14

Emma Hutchinson

Overview

This chapter explores how public health policy actions can achieve environmental and health benefits in the context of sustainable development. Action to protect the environment and human health comes from the local, national and international levels. At the local level, the actions of local or grassroots movements can have an impact on national and international policy. At the national level, public health agencies have a role in informing and influencing environmental policies, while at the international level, international environmental agreements coordinate action to reduce global environmental hazards such as climate change, biodiversity loss and stratospheric ozone depletion.

Learning objectives

By the end of this chapter you will able to:

- describe environmental policy at local, national and international levels
- appreciate the role of science in environmental decision-making
- describe activities undertaken by public health professionals to support sustainable development
- evaluate the implementation of local actions
- critically appraise progress towards the Sustainable Development Goals (SDGs)

Key terms

Agenda 21: A blueprint for sustainable development formulated at the international level for dissemination at the local level, agreed at the Rio Earth Summit in 1992.

Environmental governance: The rules, practices, policies and institutions that shape how humans interact with the environment (UNEP 2010). Good environmental governance takes into account the role of all actors that have an impact on the environment, including governments, the private sector and civil society.

> **Inter-sectoral cooperation:** Partnerships with a variety of agencies such as local authorities, NGOs and UN bodies.
>
> **International Environmental Agreements.** Series of international declarations relating to environmental concerns and sustainability.

Introduction to environmental policy for sustainable development

"Think globally, act locally".

You have seen throughout this book how humans affect the environment, and how, in turn, the environment (including the built and natural environment) affects human health. Rapid social and economic changes are causing unsustainable demands on the Earth's resources (see Chapter 3). This has led to the formulation of policy to support and promote sustainable development from the international to the local level.

Many environmental policies have an impact on public health, therefore the health sector has a role in informing environmental policy and its implementation. As discussed in Chapter 2, inter-sectoral collaboration is essential for effective public health policy. There has also been a move to participatory decision-making processes at all levels. A detailed discussion of health policy and public health governance is outside the scope of this book, but for more indepth discussion and analysis, see the *Making Health Policy* book in this series (Buse et al. 2012). In this chapter we will consider, briefly, international, national and local action, and additionally reflect on the role of science and public health in informing policy.

Action at international level

Many environmental hazards are transnational and therefore international collective action is required to address them. Examples of such international agreements to control environmental hazards include the Stockholm Convention on Persistent Organic Pollutants (see Chapter 4), the Basel Convention on the Control of Transboundary Movements of Hazardous Wastes and their Disposal (see Chapter 8), and the Convention on Transboundary Air Pollution which was implemented to control ground-level ozone (an air pollutant) (see Chapter 12).

International environmental agreements are those agreements relating to environmental concerns and sustainability which are negotiated by many governments and to which at least some countries have signed up. 'Agreement' tends to apply to bilateral or restricted multilateral treaties. A 'declaration' is a statement of intent or mutual concerns and is not always legally binding (e.g. the Rio Declaration). 'Conventions' are agreements that are not binding until sufficient countries have both signed *and* ratified them; they are usually negotiated under the auspices of an international organization.

International environmental agreements for sustainable development

Global environmental problems require international agreements because of the global scale of the problems. For example, emissions of greenhouse gases mix in the atmosphere and affect the global climate system. There are now several international agreements relating to the environment. Some of these have been discussed in previous chapters, including the Vienna Convention for the Protection of the Ozone Layer (the Montreal Protocol) (Chapter 12) and the UN Convention on Biological Diversity (UNCBD) (Chapter 13).

International agencies have an important role to play in global environmental governance (Biermann et al. 2010). The UN has been instrumental in establishing several global environmental agreements. The global perspective on sustainable development that was formalized by the UN in the Bruntland Commission in 1987 (*Our Common Future*) was followed by the Rio Earth Summit in 1992, and the World Summit for Development in 2002 where a further series of global environmental conventions and measures were initiated by the UN. In 2012, the Rio+20 Summit evaluated the progress in the 20 years since the 1992 summit and established agreed criteria for sustainable development, which formed the basis for setting the Sustainable Development Goals (SDGs). Key international environmental agreements are summarized in Table 14.1.

It is beyond the scope of this book to go into detail on any of the international accords or agreements. However, one is considered in more detail later in the chapter, the Strategic Environmental Assessment (SEA) Protocol that considers health and environment in planning. Before going into this level of detail, the next activity is designed to get you thinking more broadly about who the actors could be in promoting health in environmental agreements.

Table 14.1 Timeline of key international environmental agreements relating to sustainable development and health

Time	Event	Scientific and political context	Chapter in this book
1972	UN Conference on the Human Environment, Stockholm, marked the beginning of a comprehensive international effort to protect, preserve, and enhance the environment	The start for active international cooperation to combat acidification	

(continued)

Table 14.1 (Continued)

Time	Event	Scientific and political context	Chapter in this book
1976	Vancouver Declaration on Human Settlements mandated by the UN, further declarations in 1996 and 2001	International concern over poor urban conditions, particularly in low-income countries	
1979	Convention on Long-range Transboundary Air Pollution (CLRTAP)	Scientific demonstration of the link between sulphur emissions in continental Europe and the acidification of Scandinavian lakes	
1983	World Commission on the Environment and Development set up by the UN	To address growing concerns about the accelerating deterioration of the human environment and natural resources	Chapter 1
1985	Vienna Convention for the Protection of the Ozone Layer	Discovery of ozone hole in the stratosphere	Chapter 12
1987	*Our Common Future*, report of the World Commission on Environment and Development	Broad political concept of sustainable development was first articulated or developed	Chapters 1, 14
1987	Montreal Protocol (Convention on Substances that Deplete the Ozone Layer)	Scientific assessments by World Meteorological Organization (WMO) and UN Environment Programme (UNEP) on the health and ecological impacts of stratospheric ozone depletion	Chapter 12
1989	Basel Convention on the Control of Transboundary Movements of Hazardous Wastes and their Disposal	In response to a public outcry following the discovery, in the 1980s, in Africa and other parts of the developing world of deposits of toxic wastes imported from abroad (Secretariat of the Basel Convention 2011)	Chapter 8
1992	UN Conference on Environment and Development (Rio Earth Summit). Agenda 21 – a blueprint for sustainable development for UN member states UNCBD – UN Convention on Biological Diversity UNCCD Convention to Combat Desertification UN Framework Convention on Climate Change (UNFCCC)	1988 Intergovernmental Panel on Climate Change (IPCC) established by WMO and UNEP. Scientific assessments on the causes and impacts of climate change	Chapter 12 Chapter 14

Table 14.1 (Continued)

Time	Event	Scientific and political context	Chapter in this book
1997	Kyoto Protocol on Climate Change (subsequently ratified in 2005 by the majority of member states)	UNEP establishes a series of scientific assessments: Global Environmental Outlook (GEO) to focus on the interactions between the environment and society. GEO-1 showed that although progress had been made in confronting environmental challenges both in developing and industrial regions, the global environment had continued to degrade	
2000	UN Millennium Declaration – which then led to the Millennium Development Goals (MDGs) (global partnership to reduce extreme poverty setting out a series of time-bound targets – with a deadline of 2015)	GEO-2 concluded that continued poverty of the majority of the planet's inhabitants and excessive consumption by the minority are the two major causes of environmental degradation, and that the present course is unsustainable	Chapters 3, 14
2001	The Stockholm Convention on Persistent Organic Pollutants (subsequently came into force 2004)	A global treaty supported by scientific assessments of the health effects of peristent organic pollutants (POPs)	Chapter 4
2002	World Summit on Sustainable Development, Johannesburg, assessed progress 10 years on from Earth Summit	GEO-3 provided an overview of the main environmental developments over the previous decades, and how social, economic and other factors have contributed to the changes that have occurred	
2005	Millennium Ecosystem Assessment (MEA). Several meetings (1988–2000) led to the formation of the Millennium Assessment Steering Committee, led by UNEP	Millennium Ecosystem Assessment – scientific assessment of the condition of the world's ecosystems and implications for human health (WHO 2005)	Chapter 13
	Hyogo Framework for Action (2005–15) Building the resilience of nations and communities to disasters. A 10-year plan to make the world safer from natural hazards	HFA was endorsed by the UN General Assembly in Resolution A/RES/60/195 following the 2005 World Disaster Reduction Conference	Chapter 10

(continued)

Table 14.1 (Continued)

Time	Event	Scientific and political context	Chapter in this book
2008	WHO Commission on Social Determinants of Health, *Closing the Gap in a Generation*. The Commission included policy-makers, researchers and civil society organizations	Set up to make recommendations to governments in addressing the social factors leading to ill health and health inequities, particularly in urban areas	Chapters 1, 2, 9, 14
2009	Zagreb Declaration for Healthy Cities (by the UN)		
2010	Protocol on Strategic Environmental Assessment (UNECE 2003)		Chapter 14
2011	WHO World Conference on Social Determinants of Health, Rio Declaration on Social Determinants of Health	The recommendations of the WHO Commission on Social Determinants of Health (2008) are taken forward	Chapters 3, 9, 14
	Durban Action Plan and the Programme of Work on Protected Areas of the UNCBD	The IUCN (International Union for the Conservation of Nature) met with indigenous representatives and conservation organizations, to discuss conservation priorities in the context of indigenous rights	Chapter 13
2012	UN Rio+20 Summit (20 years on from the Earth Summit), Rio Convention on Biodiversity strategic plan 2012–20. Aichi Biodiversity Targets	'Planet Under Pressure' conference held in London in 2012, focusing on solutions to the global sustainability challenge	Chapters 1, 14
2015	UNFCCC Paris Agreement governing greenhouse gas (GHG) emissions mitigation, adaptation and finance from 2020	IPCC Fifth Assessment Report – scientific assessment of cause and impacts of climate change, 2014, 2015	Chapters 12, 13, 14
	Sendai Framework for Disaster Risk Reduction 2015–30 (UN Office for Disaster Risk Reduction – UNISDR). First major agreement of the post-2015 development agenda, with seven targets and four priorities for action United Nations Sustainable Development Summit 2015. Sustainable Development Goals (SDGs) agreed	UNISDR has science and technology platform Proposed the 2030 Agenda for Sustainable Development, with 17 time-bound SDGs	Chapter 10

Activity 14.1

Human health has been included in international environmental agreements but often not explicitly. Drawing on what you have read and learned so far in this book, which agencies should have a role in promoting health in environmental agreements? Make a list, briefly outlining your reasons.

Feedback

Previous chapters have discussed the implications for human health from climate change, air pollution and biodiversity loss. The agencies involved in promoting health in environmental agreements include:

- the WHO, which has a mandate to protect health, and also provides scientific evidence to national governments to support decision-making on international agreements for environment and health;
- international environmental agencies such as UNEP, who have a role in promoting health but also, in conjunction with the UN Development Programme (UNDP), in alleviating poverty because they provide additional justification for environmental action, and improved environmental conditions lead to improved health;
- stakeholders in international environmental policy, national governments including (e.g. the UK Department for International Development, DFID), who can influence policy-making;
- donor (funding) agencies (e.g. the World Bank, African Development Bank), who can be influential in the development field;
- regional bodies with legislative power, such as the European Union, and other regional bodies (e.g. in Africa and the Americas);
- NGOs, such as the World Wide Fund for Nature, or Oxfam, who lobby for environmental or health protection;
- civil society.

National environmental health policy

Much environmental health policy is decided at a national level. Policies and measures used to achieve environmental objectives are summarized in Table 14.2. Many actors shape national environmental policy including national and local governments, industry (individually and as members of trade organizations), NGOs (such as national wildlife groups and campaigning organizations such as Greenpeace), public health actors (such as the American Public Health Association), academics and civil society.

Table 14.2 Examples of national environmental health policies

Explicit environmental health policies	Implicit environmental health policies
Air quality standards	Urban planning
Water quality standards	Building regulations
Drinking water standards	Transport planning
Food hygiene standards	Energy production
Solid waste collection and disposal	Water resource management (e.g., reservoirs)
Regulations for toxic chemicals	Land conservation and recreation
Emissions standards	International trade and tariffs
	Agricultural pricing

Source: Modified from Frumkin (2010)

Understanding their respective motivations helps to explain particular policy choices (Frumkin 2010).

Some environmental policies and laws are based directly on avoiding negative health outcomes (Table 14.2). For example, the US EPA's ambient air quality standards are set at levels required to protect public health (Frumkin 2010). Well intended environmental policies may also have unforeseen consequences. For example, the widespread use of pesticides has increased agricultural yields but these chemicals have had detrimental effects on ecosystems and human health. Balancing the need for action with the need for caution over policy actions is a difficult judgement faced by policy-makers.

Links between national and international policy

International environmental agreements have been instrumental in developing national policies in many countries. Countries belonging to the European Union have had additional impetus from EU directives informing policy and in needing to achieve legal compliance with these directives. A directive is a legislative act of the European Union, which requires member states to achieve a particular result without dictating the means of achieving that result. For example, in the area of pollution control from transport, in order to comply with Directive 91/441/EEC (the Consolidated Emissions Directive), the fitting of vehicle exhaust catalysts became mandatory on all new light petrol vehicles from 1993 in the UK (AA 2014).

The role of science in national policy

Having considered some examples of environmental policies, it is useful to think about how science can be used to inform environmental decision-making. Few disagree that science should inform policy, however, it is not the only consideration, as decision-makers need also to consider equity issues, politics, costs (social and economic), and also cultural and religious traditions.

Health impact assessments (HIAs) are used to quantify the amount of disease caused by environmental risks or policies (see examples in Chapters 4 and 7 on chemicals and air pollution and Chapter 11 on energy). The WHO, among others, recommends that such a quantified estimate of an environmental impact on a population should be a part of decision-making for setting policies or defining protective measures, and also be used for public information (WHO 2012a).

Large-scale scientific assessments have been used in the formation of international agreements such as the UN Framework Convention on Climate Change (UNFCCC) which uses the findings of comprehensive assessments from the Intergovernmental Panel on Climate Change (IPCC) (Table 14.1).

Strategic environmental assessment (the SEA protocol)

Historically, environmental impact assessments (EIAs) for plans and projects focused on the impacts on the physical and biological environment. The Protocol on Strategic Environmental Assessment (the SEA Protocol) attempts to improve the process by placing a special emphasis on human health (London Declaration on Action in Partnership: UNECE 2003, 2010). A general definition of strategic environmental assessment is the formalized, systematic and comprehensive process of evaluating the environmental impacts of a policy, plan or programme and its alternatives, including the preparation of a written report on the findings of that evaluation, and using the findings in publicly accountable decision-making (Thérivel et al. 1992).

SEA allows the identification and prevention of possible environmental impact at the outset of planning and programme design, at the decision-making stage. An example of this might be to develop a more sustainable transport policy rather than just minimizing the environmental impact of building a road, the traditional place of environmental impact assessment. It also enables the environmental objectives to be considered on a par with socioeconomic ones, allowing better integration of sustainable development.

The aim of this protocol is to provide for a high level of protection of the environment, including health, by:

- ensuring that environmental considerations, including health, are thoroughly taken into account in the development of plans and programmes;
- contributing to the consideration of environmental and health concerns in the elaboration of policies and legislation;
- establishing clear, transparent and effective procedures for strategic environmental assessment;

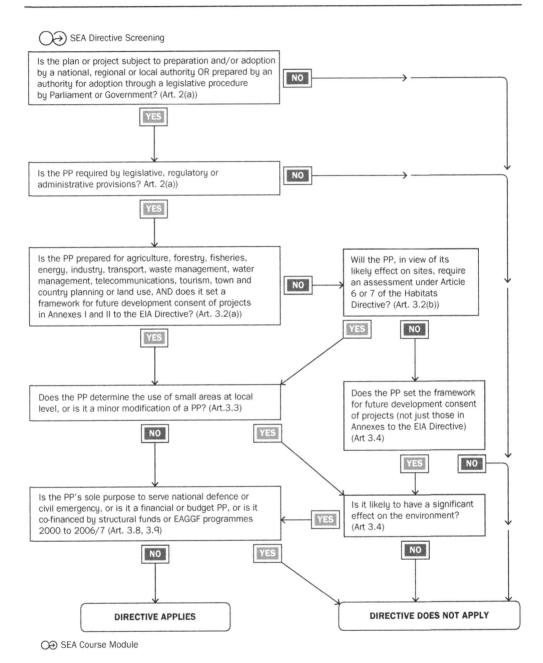

Figure 14.1 SEA directive screening.

Source: http://sea.unu.edu/course/wp-gallery/SEA_directive.pdf

- providing for public participation in strategic environmental assessment;
- integrating environmental and health concerns into measures and instruments designed to further sustainable development.

There is a special emphasis on health throughout the protocol. However, a review of strategic environmental assessments (SEAs) in Scotland found that health was not consistently considered in policies, and recommended that there was a role for a greater involvement of the health sector in scoping of health issues in these assessments, and that this may enhance their quality (Douglas et al. 2011).

The protocol defines procedures that need to be followed and it places a special emphasis on public participation, as well as on consultation with authorities. It was mandated in 2010: the SEA Directive requires SEAs for those plans and programmes that meet a complex set of screening requirements, as shown in Figure 14.1.

SEA addresses some of the limitations of EIA, such as a narrow focus and limited range of alternatives and mitigation measures, reactionary nature, assessment of direct impacts, and is better able to address a wider range of alternatives and mitigation measures and assess a broader range of impacts, such as cumulative, global, secondary and synergistic impacts because it:

- incorporates environmental issues into project planning and decision-making;
- considers alternatives or mitigation measures beyond project level; and
- involves consultation on more strategic issues (UNU 2006).

 Activity 14.2

You are a public health representative on a committee set up to ensure a SEA is carried out on a programme for creating a series of microdams in your area. The affected area is currently agricultural land and pristine forest; the dam will provide electricity, be stocked with fish and water will be channelled for irrigation downstream. What will you need to include in your report?

Feedback

These are some of the issues you would have brought before the committee.

- The environmental and health consequences. The advantages include: provision of electricity, irrigation, local jobs and flood control. The disadvantages include: loss of agricultural land, enviromental and health issues associated with construction including transport of material to site, loss of biodiversity with loss of forest, risk of disaster if dam collapsed, water restriction to communities downstream, risk of water- and vector-borne diseases.

- Clear, transparent and effective procedures for SEA should be established and monitored.
- Public participation should occur, i.e. all communities affected need to be fairly consulted, including those communities living downstream of the proposed dam.
- Sustainable development should be considered, i.e. does this project meet the needs of the current local population without jeopardizing others? The impact of carbon reduction from changed energy production should also be considered.

Local government and civil society

Policies can also arise from local needs and concerns. 'Grassroots' policy relies on local individuals or groups coming together to express their concerns for a change in policy or action on environmental health in their area. The repercussions of such actions can inform and influence national policy, or remain as local initiatives (addressed by local government) – for instance, a community association lobbying for better housing conditions or a clean water supply. The multiplication of many such local initiatives can also have an effect on the global environment.

Implementation of sustainable development at the local level

Having considered the roles of international agencies, national and local government and local action, the following section discusses and describes Agenda 21, a blueprint for sustainable development formulated at the international level for dissemination at the local level, which cuts across all these sectors.

Agenda 21

Agenda 21 sets out a global action plan for sustainable development. In order to integrate environmental concerns into development, Agenda 21 relies on the cooperation of government (at all levels), non-governmental agencies (e.g. health, industry, education, charities, etc.) and local communities, and that the various agencies, both UN and other, do not work in isolation but cooperate in inter-sector collaboration for the most effective responses. One of the most important precepts of Agenda 21 is the involvement of local representatives in initiating and implementing regional policies that will promote development while maintaining a healthy environment.

The implementation of Agenda 21 is intended to involve action at international, national, regional and local levels. Some national and state governments have legislated or advised that local authorities take steps to implement the plan locally, as many of the issues have their problems and solutions rooted in local activities, and the participation and cooperation of local authorities will play a critical role in the fulfilment of Agenda 21's objectives.

Putting ideas into action

There are a number of ongoing activities related to the achievement of Agenda 21 objectives throughout the world, such as the WHO 'Healthy Cities' movement and the 'Sustainable Cities' movement (UNCHS). A review of Agenda 21 (UN-DESA 2012) concluded that progress has been limited, with three areas (changing consumption patterns, promoting sustainable human settlement development, protection of the atmosphere) regarded as having made no progress, while five areas (involvement of NGOs and local authorities; science for sustainable development; international institutional arrangements; international legal instruments; international mechanisms and policy) were considered to have made good progress. Areas that need addressing include sustainable consumption and production – global consumption has increased, remaining high in high-income countries, but also increasing in emerging economies such as China and Brazil. While there have been some good examples of progressive urban policy, inequalities and poor environmental conditions remain in many urban areas in high-, middle- and low-income countries, and slum populations are still rising.

Although the implementation of Agenda 21 remains incomplete, there are some examples of good practice, one of which is outlined below.

Box 14.1:   Example of good practice – Local Agenda 21

The following extract is about the implementation of Agenda 21 in Peru (ICLEI, IDRC and UNEP 1996).

The Provincial Municipality of Cajamarca, Peru. Participatory regional development planning and inter-institutional consensus-building for a sustainable development plan

Background The Provincial Municipality of Cajamarca, located in the high altitude sierra of northern Peru, is a local government authority with jurisdiction over the entire province, including both urban and rural areas. Approximately 55% of Cajamarca's 233,575 residents live in rural areas.

The provincial capital, Cajamarca City, serves as a commercial center for the activities of the surrounding countryside. The province's main economic activities include agriculture and livestock production, followed by commerce, mining, and tourism. Residents lack basic services and many rural citizens live in extreme poverty.

The development planning issues faced by the municipality of Cajamarca illustrate the inter-dependency between urban and rural development and the need for coordinated planning. Small and large scale cattle ranching and agricultural production are the predominant economic activities in rural areas. Increased demand for milk and milk products has resulted in cattle farmers encroaching on marginal lands prone to environmental degradation. The region's watershed has been seriously affected. Deforestation, soil erosion, reduced water quality and quantity, and the loss of biodiversity have been the results. Due to increasing population and unemployment in rural areas, people have migrated to provincial urban centers in unprecedented numbers. Consequently, municipalities such as Cajamarca have experienced unplanned growth. Squatter settlements have emerged in areas that are fertile and unsuitable for housing development.

Increased demand for basic services has severely undermined the municipal government's ability to manage and deliver quality services. The Kilish River, the main source of drinking water, was contaminated from rural mining activities and a lack of sewerage. Water-borne diseases afflict the population. Poor management of storm water run-off in urban areas persistently results in flooding problems. The regional level of government traditionally has authority over development in Peru, while public and private institutions deliver development infrastructure and services at local levels. Private institutions such as corporations, government agencies, and NGOs have primary responsibility for agrarian issues such as forestation and agricultural management, while both private and public sector institutions are involved with health and education issues, among others. Public sector institutions have extremely limited budgets, while private institutions have outside funding. Lack of coordination between these institutions in Cajamarca resulted in the duplication of services and uneven resource allocation between urban and rural areas.

Program Description In accordance with Agenda 21, the municipality of Cajamarca decided to implement a participatory regional development planning process designed to coordinate development activities and improve the delivery of community services.

Inter-Institutional Consensus-Building The Provincial Council established new partnership structures . . . which for the first time convened a wide range of stakeholders, including several private and public institutions operating in rural and urban affairs, local communities, farmers, entrepreneurs, and state and national governing organizations. The initiative, known as the "Inter-Institutional Consensus-Building Process," aimed for broad-based consensus on projects that would form the basis of a Provincial Sustainable Development Plan.

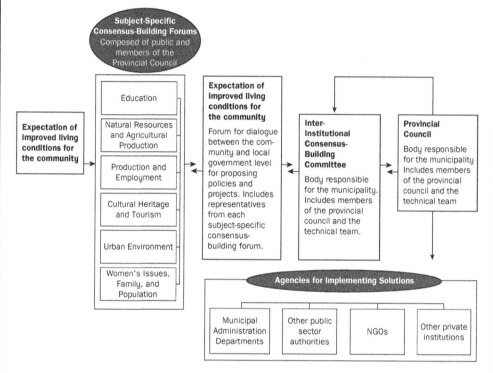

Figure 14.2 Inter-institutional consensus-building in Cajamarca, Peru.
Source: ICLEI, IDRC, UNEP (1996).

Several initiatives aimed at promoting sustainable agriculture and urban settlements and improving environmental and health conditions were implemented; for example, a permanent health package for Cajamarca City, a refuse collection program, and a parks and gardens improvement program responsible for the sowing of more than 80,000 seedlings along streets and in parks.

Since this time, it has been reported that natural resource management has improved significantly in Cajamarca with the implementation of this participatory governance structure (ICLEI 2007). The key instrument for coordinated planning was the 'mesas de concertación' or inter-institutional consensus building related to resource allocation and use. This brought together different levels of government, district mayors, NGOs, the local mining company, and other business interests to discuss development priorities and negotiate a sustainable development plan. This approach presents a unique working model of a more participatory and open approach to planning, one that defines sustainability and equity as central objectives.

The role of public health in sustainable development

There has been growing recognition of the relationship of public health with the environment and sustainable development (Adshead et al. 2006; Hanlon and Carlisle 2008). Previous chapters have described the adverse effects on human health from unsustainable development (through unplanned urbanization, climate change and biodiversity loss). Action to achieve sustainable development has co-benefits for health, and as such, public health actors have a role in promoting sustainable development through improved public health.

As we have seen in previous chapters, sustainable development and health are closely interrelated in several ways (UNCED 1992; WHO 1992):

- first, the concept of sustainable development embraces environmental, social and economic dimensions and aspires to health-enhancing communities, societies and environments;
- second, health is determined by a range of environmental, social and economic influences, and therefore the health of people, places and the planet are interdependent;
- third, the causes and consequences of unsustainable development and poor health are interrelated and frequently pose further challenges.

The underlying causes of common chronic diseases are inextricably linked to our dependence on a plentiful supply of energy from fossil fuels and high levels of consumption. The solutions not only offer the avoidance of negative effects but actively open up new opportunities into the future, for policy, industry and communities. For example, promoting walking and cycling in urban areas in place of driving reduces not only traffic emissions and therefore air pollution, but also obesity and traffic accidents, and improves cardiovascular health (as discussed in Chapters 7 and 9). It has been suggested that reduction of carbon emissions should be a public health strategy (Bloomberg and Aggarwala 2008). Fast growing economies such as India and China are increasingly facing the chronic health problems of high-income countries such as obesity, cardiovascular and respiratory disease. As their wealth grows, in the absence of effective international or national legislation, they may respond to civil pressure to improve public health and see that a focus on sustainable development, in particular low carbon development, will lead to such an improvement.

Health practitioners have a crucial and distinctive role to play in influencing public opinion and the policies of national and international governments and agencies, by triggering collective support for action using the weight of scientific evidence on health (Gill and Stott 2009; Haines et al. 2009). There are three special characteristics of the health argument for sustainable development, comprising: action towards sustainable development should be implemented anyway for good public health reasons (health benefits argument – in that action to ensure sustainable development has the added co-benefit of improving health, e.g. ensuring access to adequate and clean water); the content of the health-based argument – which is based on positive language – such as improved quality of life and social justice, and the short time in which effects of personal action can be realized at the personal level; and the force with which they can be delivered to governments and electorates.

 Activity 14.3

What are the main challenges in achieving sustainable development and health improvement? How do they differ in low-, middle- and high-income countries? Think about how change can be implemented.

Feedback

Your answers should consider:

- the necessity to balance economic growth with environmental protection;
- the impact of the type of economy in each country (e.g. energy use/ technological societies, carbon-intensive economies) – these all tend to be factors associated with unsustainable development and inequitable use of resources;
- the impact of national policy, legislation, environmental standards and enforcement;
- the underlying health burden and resulting priorities for governments – environmental standards tend to be less stringent in areas where there are also higher health burdens due to a lack of governance or technical capacity;
- a lack of awareness on environment and health issues in the general public and in decision-makers.

The challenges may vary between countries. For middle-income countries, rapid economic growth and the associated increase in carbon-intense economies may be associated with increases in personal wealth.

Requirements for the implementation of change include consultation, collaboration, clear planning and setting of objectives, and measures for evaluating effectiveness. Implementation should incorporate social justice and equitable economic development.

Pathways to sustainable development

In 2000, the Millennium Development goals (MDGs) were established to attempt to combat poverty, hunger, disease, illiteracy, environmental degradation and discrimination against women, as described in Chapter 2.

Significant progress has been made in achieving the MDGs, and a number of targets have been met: reducing extreme poverty by half; reducing the

Table 14.3 Sustainable Development Goals (SDGs)

Goal	Aim
1 Poverty	End poverty in all its forms everywhere
2 Hunger	End hunger, achieve food security and improved nutrition and promote sustainable agriculture
3 Health	Ensure healthy lives and promote wellbeing for all at all ages
4 Education	Ensure inclusive and quality education for all and promote lifelong learning
5 Equality	Achieve gender equality and empower all women and girls
6 Sanitation	Ensure access to water and sanitation for all
7 Affordable and clean energy	Ensure access to affordable, reliable, sustainable and modern energy for all
8 Economic growth	Promote inclusive and sustainable economic growth, employment and decent work for all
9 Infrastructure, industrialization	Build resilient infrastructure, promote sustainable industrialization and foster innovation
10 Reduced inequalities	Reduce inequality within and among countries
11 Sustainable cities and community	Make cities inclusive, safe, resilient and sustainable
12 Responsible production and consumption	Ensure sustainable consumption and production patterns
13 Climate action	Take urgent action to combat climate change and its impacts
14 Life below water	Conserve and sustainably use the oceans, seas and marine resources
15 Life on land	Sustainably manage forests, combat desertification, halt and reverse land degradation, halt biodiversity loss
16 Peace, justice and strong institutions	Promote just, peaceful and inclusive societies
17 Partnership for the goals	Revitalize the global partnership for sustainable development

Source: UN (2016)

number of people without access to improved drinking water sources by half (see Chapter 5); improving the lives of at least 100 million slum dwellers (see Chapter 9); and gender equality in access to primary education. There have also been improvements in reducing child and maternal mortality, a decline in HIV infections (although this varies across regions and countries) and a reduction in malaria. However, the achievements of the MDGs have been uneven across and within regions and countries with the poorest and those most marginalized and discriminated against on the basis of gender, age, disability and ethnicity seeing the least progress. Hunger and under-nutrition remain critical, and progress on environmental goals is poor. Violence has become one of the largest obstacles to development, with approximately one-fifth of humanity residing in countries experiencing political conflict. The MDGs have been criticized for focusing on addressing income differentials rather than inequality and inequity in wider areas.

The focus of the post-2015 UN development agenda is sustainable development, based on the premises of inclusive social development, environmental sustainability, inclusive economic development, and peace and security (UN General Assembly 2012; WHO 2012b). Seventeen goals have been agreed that cover these areas of concern (UN-DESA 2015) (see Table 14.3).

Each goal has several specific targets and indicators (169 targets in total) that need to be achieved by 2020 or 2030. Unlike the MDGs, the SDGs apply to all countries (high-, middle- and low-income).

The SDGs are interdependent, and many of them encompass important determinants of health (such as energy, sustainable cities, climate change, equality, etc.). Health is also a factor in achieving the goals. For example, better health enables children to learn and adults to undertake employment. Gender equality is essential to the achievement of better health. Reducing poverty, hunger and environmental degradation positively influences, but also depends on, better health (WHO 2012b).

Summary

In this chapter you have learned how health, environment and sustainable development concerns inform local, national and global policy. International agreements are central to global environmental policy, however there are often difficulties in achieving consensus between countries and implementation within countries. National policy-making and action also play a role in ensuring the minimizing of environmental damage and the maximizing of health benefits, and the integration of economic, social and environmental concerns. The aspiration for sustainable development and environmental equity has informed the principles of Agenda 21, and its promotion of community-based enterprises directed at improving local health and environments. Partnership working and inclusive and sustainable development have been recognized as the way forward.

References

AA (2014) Euro emissions standards, https://www.theaa.com/motoring_advice/fuels-and-environment/euro-emissions-standards.html, accessed 29 September 2015.

Adshead, F., Thorpe, A. and Rutter, J. (2006) Sustainable development and public health: a national perspective, *Public Health*, 120: 1102–5.

Biermann, F. et al. (2010) Earth system governance: a research framework, *International Environmental Agreements*, 10: 277–98.

Bloomberg, M.R. and Aggarwala, R.T. (2008) Think locally, act globally: how curbing global warming emissions can improve local public health, *American Journal of Preventive Medicine*, 35(5): 414–23.

Buse, K., Mays, N. and Walt, G. (2012) *Making Health Policy*. Maidenhead: Open University Press.

Douglas, M.J., Carver, H. and Katikireddi, S.V. (2011) How well do strategic environmental assessments in Scotland consider human health?, *Public Health*, 125: 585–91.

Frumkin, H. (ed.) (2010) *Environmental Health: from global to local*. San Francisco: Jossey-Bass.

Gill, M. and Stott, R. (2009) Leadership: how to influence national and international policy, in J. Griffiths et al. (eds) *The Health Practitioner's Guide to Climate Change: diagnosis and cure*. London: Earthscan.

Haines, A. et al. (2009) Public health benefits of strategies to reduce greenhouse-gas emissions: overview and implications for policy makers, *Lancet*, 374: 2104–14.

Hanlon, P. and Carlisle, S. (2008) Do we face a third revolution in human history? If so, how will public health respond?, *Journal of Public Health*, 30(4): 355–61.

ICLEI (2007) Natural resource management improves in Cajamarca, http://www.iclei.org/details/article/natural-resource-management-improves-in-cajamarca.html, accessed 10 February 2013.

ICLEI, IDRC, UNEP (1996) *The Local Agenda Planning Guide: an Introduction to sustainable development planning*. Canada: ICLEI/IDRC.

Secretariat of the Basel Convention (2011) Overview, http://www.basel.int/TheConvention/Overview/tabid/1271/Default.aspx, accessed 29 September 2015.

Thérivel, R., Wilson, E., Thompson, S., Heaney, D. and Pritchard, D. (1992) *Strategic Environmental Assessment*. London: Earthscan Publications.

UN (2016) *Sustainable Development Goals: 17 goals to transform our world*, http://www.un.org/sustainabledevelopment/, accessed 21 January 2016.

UN General Assembly (2012) *Annual report of the Secretary-General: accelerating progress towards the Millennium Development Goals – options for sustained and inclusive growth and issues for advancing the United Nations development agenda beyond 2015* (August), http://www.un.org/en/development/desa/policy/untaskteam_undf/sgreport.pdf, accessed 11 December 2012.

UN-DESA (Department of Economic and Social Affairs) (2015) *Sustainable Development Goals*, https://sustainabledevelopment.un.org/topics, accessed 29 September 2015.

UN-DESA (Department of Economic and Social Affairs) (2012) *Review of implementation of Agenda 21 and the Rio Principles: synthesis*, http://sustainabledevelopment.un.org/content/documents/641Synthesis_report_Web.pdf, accessed 11 December 2012.

UNCED (1992) United Nations Conference on Environment and Development, Rio de Janeiro, https://sustainabledevelopment.un.org/milestones/unced, accessed 26 January 2017.

UNECE (2003) *The SEA (Kyiv) Protocol*, http://www.unece.org/env/eia/sea_protocol.html, accessed 11 July 2013.

UNECE (2010) *SEA Protocol*, http://www.unece.org/env/eia.

UNEP (2010) Environmental governance: six priority area factsheets, http://www.unep.org/pdf/brochures/EnvironmentalGovernance.pdf, accessed 10 February 2013.

UNU (2006) Strategic environmental assessment: course module, http://sea.unu.edu/course/?page_id=30, accessed 18 March 2013.

WHO (1992) *Our Planet, Our Health*. Geneva: WHO.

WHO (2005) *Ecosystems and Human Well-being: health synthesis*. Geneva: WHO, http://www.who.int/globalchange/ecosystems/en/, accessed 3 May 2016.

WHO (2012a) *Quantifying Environmental Health Impacts*, http://www.who.int/quantifying_ehimpacts/en/, accessed 11 December 2012.

WHO (2012b) *Social Determinants of Health*, http://www.who.int/topics/social_determinants/en/, accessed 11 December 2012.

Glossary

Acclimatization: The physiological and behavioural adaptation to climatic variation.

Active transport: Modes of transport that involve physical activity, such as walking or cycling.

Adaptation: (in relation to climate change) Adjustment in natural or human systems in response to actual or expected climatic stimuli or their effects, which moderates harm or exploits beneficial opportunities.

Anthropocene: An informal geologic chronological term that serves to mark the period of time when human activities have had a significant global impact on the Earth's systems.

Anthropogenic: Caused or made by human activity.

Best Practical Environmental Option (BPEO): Identifies the preferred waste route in order to minimize harm and ensure the protection of the environment.

Bioaccumulation: Storage of a stable substance in living tissues, resulting in a much higher concentration than in the environment.

Biodiversity: Variability among living organisms including the variability within and between species and within and between ecosystems.

Biofuel: A type of fuel whose energy is derived from biological carbon fixation, for example, bioethanol and biodiesel.

Biomagnification: Increase in the concentration of a substance through the food chain, i.e. from prey to predator (presupposes bioaccumulation).

Biomass fuel: Energy from organic material, such as animal dung, wood or crop residues.

Carbon sink: A natural or artificial reservoir that accumulates and stores carbon-containing compounds for an indefinite period. The process by which carbon sinks remove carbon dioxide (CO_2) from the atmosphere is known as carbon sequestration.

Carbon-neutral: Property of fuel or product if the same amount of carbon emissions are released from its combustion or production as are later absorbed from the atmosphere.

Climate change: Refers to any change in climate over time, whether due to natural variability or as a result of human activity. The United Nations Framework Convention on Climate Change (UNFCCC) defines 'climate change' as a 'change of climate which is attributed directly or indirectly to human activity that alters the composition of the global atmosphere and which is in addition to natural climate variability observed over comparable time periods'.

Climate scenarios: Plausible and self-consistent descriptions of the future global climate but have used different assumptions and have uncertainties in their estimates.

Climate variability: Refers to variations in the mean state and other statistics (such as standard deviations, statistics of extremes, etc.) of the climate on all temporal and spatial scales beyond that of individual weather events. Variability may be due to natural internal processes within the climate system (internal variability), or to variations in natural or anthropogenic external forcing (external variability).

Co-benefits (also called ancillary benefits): Benefits to health that may accrue from policies or programmes implemented for other (non-health) reasons.

Composting: The biological process of breaking up of organic waste into a humus-like substance by various micro-organisms.

Demographic transition: The transition from high to low birth rate (and mortality rates) in a population.

DPSEEA: Framework for describing the influences of the environment on health (D drivers, P pressures, S states, E exposures, E effects, A actions).

Driving forces: Factors that create the circumstances in which environmental health conditions develop or increase environmental hazards. They can also be described as distal causes of ill health in a population.

Ecological footprint: Measures the amount of renewable and non-renewable ecologically productive land area required to support the resource demands and absorb the wastes of a given population or specific activities.

Ecosystem: The interactive system formed from all living organisms and their abiotic (physical and chemical) environment within a given area. Ecosystems cover a hierarchy of spatial scales and can comprise the entire globe, biomes at the continental scale or small, well-circumscribed systems such as a small pond.

Ecosystem services: Ecological processes or functions having monetary or non-monetary value to individuals or society at large, which include (1) supporting services such as productivity or biodiversity maintenance, (2) provisioning services such as food, fibre, or fish, (3) regulating services such as climate regulation or carbon sequestration, and (4) cultural services such as tourism or spiritual and aesthetic appreciation.

El Niño Southern Oscillation (ENSO): A climate phenomenon that includes warming of the ocean surface off the western coast of South America that occurs every 4 to 12 years.

Emissions: Any form of pollution that is discharged into the environment.

Energy ladder: A model of household energy use whereby increasing income is associated with the household shifting to cleaner and more efficient energy sources (and movement up the energy ladder).

Environmental governance: Environmental governance comprises the rules, practices, policies and institutions that shape how humans interact with the environment. Good environmental governance takes into account the role of all actors that impact the environment, including governments, NGOs, the private sector and civil society.

Environmental justice: the fair distribution of environmental benefits and burdens and the fair treatment and meaningful participation of all people, regardless of race, ethnicity, income, national origin or educational level in the decision-making processes.

Environmental risk transition: Changing patterns of environmental hazards in a population associated with economic development.

Epidemiological transition: Changing patterns of disease in a population, from high burdens to infectious diseases and malnutrition to increased incidence of non-communicable diseases. It is closely associated with the demographic transition.

Externalities: Social benefits and costs that are not included in the market price of an economic good.

Food security: Physical and economic access for everyone and at all times to enough foods that are nutritious, safe, personally acceptable and culturally appropriate, produced and distributed in ways that are environmentally sound and just.

Fracking: See **hydraulic fracturing**.

Fuel poverty: A situation in which householders would have to spend a high proportion of their income on heating and other fuel costs to keep adequately warm at reasonable cost, given their income. In the UK, fuel poverty is now defined as occurring when a household's required fuel costs are above the national median level, and at that level of expenditure the household would be left with a residual income below the official poverty line.

Global environmental change: Environmental changes that affect global systems, including climate change, biodiversity loss and land use change.

Globalization: A set of processes that are changing the nature of human interaction by intensifying interactions across certain boundaries that have hitherto served to separate individuals and population groups. These spatial, temporal and cognitive boundaries have been increasingly eroded, resulting in new forms of social organization and interaction across these boundaries.

Green infrastructure: The network of multifunctional green space which supports natural and ecological processes and is integral to the health and quality of life of sustainable communities.

Green space: An area of grass, trees, or other vegetation set apart for recreational or aesthetic purposes or for the control of hazards (e.g. natural flood management) in an otherwise urban environment.

Greenhouse gas: Greenhouse gases are gaseous constituents of the atmosphere, both natural and anthropogenic, that absorb and emit radiation at specific wavelengths within the spectrum of infrared radiation emitted by the Earth's surface, the atmosphere, and clouds. This property causes the greenhouse effect. Water vapour (H_2O), carbon dioxide (CO_2), nitrous oxide (N_2O), methane (CH_4) and ozone (O_3) are the primary greenhouse gases in the Earth's atmosphere.

Hazardous waste: Waste that poses substantial or potential threats to public health or the environment. In the USA, hazardous waste has a legal definition as it is subject to formal regulation.

Health impact assessment (HIA): A means of assessing the health impacts of policies, plans and projects in diverse economic sectors using quantitative, qualitative and participatory techniques.

Healthy city: A healthy community in which all systems work well (and work together), and in which all citizens enjoy a good quality of life. This means that the health of the community is affected by the social and environmental determinants of health and development – the factors that influence individual and community health and development.

Hydraulic fracturing (fracking): Method of gas extraction that involves drilling a well shaft into the rock and pumping in water and chemicals to open cracks that will release the gas.

Infrastructure: The basic facilities, services and installations needed for the functioning of a community, such as transport and communication systems, water and power lines, schools, post offices and prisons.

Life-cycle analysis: An assessment approach that ensures that all stages in a fuel's life cycle are considered. It is sometimes called a 'cradle to grave' approach.

Mitigation: (climate change) An intervention to reduce the anthropogenic climate change or other environmental hazard. For example, strategies to reduce greenhouse gas emissions and enhance greenhouse gas sinks.

Obesogenic environment: An environment where factors play an important role in determining both nutrition and physical activity leading to increased obesity. Environmental factors may operate by determining the availability and consumption of different foodstuffs and the levels of physical activity undertaken by populations.

Peri-urban: On the urban margins.

Polluter pays principle: Principle that the party responsible for producing pollution is responsible for paying for the damage done to the natural environment.

Precautionary principle: A principle that advocates the use of prudent social policy in the absence of comprehensive empirical evidence in an attempt to solve a problem.

Proximity principle: Principle that *waste* should be treated and disposed of close to where it was produced.

Psycho-social: Relating to the interrelation of social factors and individual thought and behaviour.

Renewable energy: Energy sources that do not deplete, or are naturally replenished after use.

Risk transition: The process by which societies move from exposure to traditional hazards to exposure to modern hazards.

Scenario: A plausible and often simplified description of how the future may develop, based on a coherent and internally consistent set of assumptions about driving forces and key relationships.

Stratosphere: The layer of the atmosphere above the troposphere.

Stratospheric ozone depletion: Reduction of ozone in the stratosphere.

Sustainable development: Meeting the needs of the present generation without compromising the ability of future generations to meet their needs.

Tolerable daily intake: An estimate of the daily intake of a substance which can occur over a lifetime without appreciable health risk

Transboundary air pollutant: A pollutant that originates in one country but is able to cause damage in another country's environment, by crossing borders through pathways like water or air.

Transnational: (as opposed to international) Refers to transborder flows that largely circumvent national borders and can thus be beyond the control of national governments alone.

Troposphere: The lowest part of the atmosphere from the surface to about 10 km in altitude in mid-latitudes (ranging from 9 km in high latitudes to 16 km in the tropics on average) where clouds and 'weather' phenomena occur. In the troposphere, temperatures generally decrease with height.

Urban planning: A technical and political process concerned with the control of the use of land and design of the urban environment, including transportation networks, to guide and ensure the orderly development of settlements and communities

Urban transition: Increasing proportion of nation's population living in urban areas

Urbanization: Increasing concentration of people and economic activities in towns and cities.

Waste hierarchy: Methods of waste disposal from reduce (best environmental option) to disposal (worst).

Water stress: An area experiences water stress when annual water resources drop below 1,700 m^3 per person per year for meeting total water requirements, including agriculture, industry, energy, and the environment.

Index

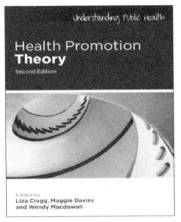

HEALTH PROMOTION THEORY
Second Edition

Liza Cragg, Maggie Davies and Wendy Macdowall

9780335263202 (Paperback)
October 2013

eBook also available

Part of the *Understanding Public Health* series, this book offers students and practitioners an accessible exploration of the origins and development of health promotion. It highlights the philosophical, ethical and political debates that influence health promotion today while also explaining the theories, frameworks and methodologies that help us understand public health problems and develop effective health promotion responses.

Key features:

- Offers more in-depth coverage of key determinants of health and how these interact with health promotion
- Revised structure to allow more depth of coverage of health promotion theory
- Updated material and case examples that reflect contemporary health promotion challenges

www.openup.co.uk

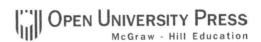

OPEN UNIVERSITY PRESS
McGraw - Hill Education

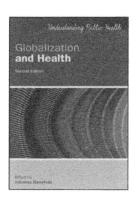

Globalization and Health
2nd Edition

Johanna Hanefeld

ISBN: 978-0-335-26408-7 (Paperback)
eBook: 978-0-335-26409-4
2015

Global health is a relatively new but rapidly expanding field as public health practitioners recognize the important challenges that global changes are posing for human health. Health issues are increasingly crossing national boundaries, and this book explores the actors that shape global health and explores some of the key issues in global health.

Key topics include:

- Social change linked to globalization
- Governance of global health
- Pharmaceuticals and tobacco

www.openup.co.uk

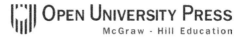

OPEN UNIVERSITY PRESS
McGraw - Hill Education

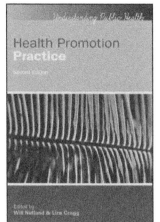

Health Promotion Practice
2nd edition

Will Nutland and Liza Cragg

ISBN: 9780335264063 (Paperback)
eBook: 9780335264070
2015

This fully revised text offers students and practitioners a grounding in the practice of health promotion and introduces a range of methods that are used in health promotion practice. It also helps to develop skills needed to do health promotion in a range of settings, including project management, partnership working, needs assessment and evaluation. Whether the public health intervention is through face to face contact with individuals, or is community based, or involves strategic policy development, this book now also explores recent developments such as in social media and web based health promotion interventions.

This second edition:

- provides practical guidance and tools for planning, delivering and evaluating health promotion
- gives greater emphasis to upstream health promotion interventions, including Healthy Public Policy and health advocacy
- includes activities to help you make applications to your own study or practice of health promotion

www.mheducation.co.uk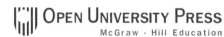